THE HEART OF YOGA

OSHO

Extemporaneous talks given by Osho at the
OSHO International Meditation Resort, Pune, India

the heart of **Yoga**

How to Become More Beautiful and Happy

YOGA: THE SCIENCE OF THE SOUL

OSHO

The book is Volume 2 of a ten-part series of talks by Osho, commenting on the
Yoga Sutras of Patajali: *Yoga: The Science of the Soul*, given to a live audience. All
of Osho's talks have been published in full as books, and are also available as
original audio recordings. Audio recordings and the complete text archive can be
found via the online OSHO Library at www.osho.com/library

OSHO and OSHO Vision are registered trademarks of OSHO International
Foundation
www.osho.com/trademarks

OSHO MEDIA INTERNATIONAL
New York – Zurich – Mumbai
an imprint of
OSHO INTERNATIONAL
www.osho.com/oshointernational

Distributed by Publishers Group Worldwide
www.pgw.com

Library of Congress Catalog-In-Publication Data is available

Printed in USA by Bang Printing

ISBN: 978-1-938755-72-9
This title is also available in eBook format ISBN: 978-0-88050-087-6

Contents

Preface

Patanjali – I call him the scientist of the religious world, the mathematician of mysticism, the logician of the illogical. Two opposites meet in him. If a scientist reads Patanjali's *Yoga Sutras* he will understand immediately. A Wittgenstein, a logical mind, will immediately feel an affinity with Patanjali. He's absolutely logical. And if he leads you toward the illogical, he leads you in such logical steps you never know when he has left the logic and taken you beyond it.

He moves like a philosopher, a thinker, and makes such subtle distinctions that the moment he takes you into *nirvichara*, into no-contemplation, you will not be able to see when the jump has been taken. He has cut the jump into many small steps.

With Patanjali you will never feel fear, because he knows where you will feel fear. He cuts the steps smaller and smaller, almost as if you move on the plain ground. He takes you so slowly that you cannot observe when the jump has happened, when you have crossed the boundary. And he is also a poet, a mystic – a very rare combination.

There are mystics like Tilopa, there are great poets like the *rishis* of the Upanishads, there are great logicians like Aristotle, but you cannot find a Patanjali. He is such a combination that since him there has been no one who can be compared to him. It is very easy to be a poet because you are out of one piece. It is very easy to be a logician – you are made of one piece. It is almost impossible to be a Patanjali because you comprehend so many opposites – and he combines them all in such a beautiful harmony. That's why he has become the alpha and the omega of the whole tradition of Yoga.

In fact, it was not he who invented Yoga; Yoga is far more ancient. Yoga had been there for many centuries before Patanjali. He is not the discoverer, but he almost became the discoverer and founder just because of this rare combination of his personality. Many people had worked before him and almost everything was known, but Yoga was waiting for a Patanjali. And suddenly, when Patanjali spoke about it, everything fell in line and he became the founder. He was not the founder, but his personality is such a combination of opposites, he comprehends in himself such incomprehensible elements, he became the founder – almost the founder. Now Yoga will always be associated with Patanjali.

Osho
Yoga: The Science of the Soul, Vol. 3

1

The Meaning of Samadhi

Sampragyata samadhi is the samadhi that is
accompanied by reasoning, reflection, bliss, and a
sense of pure being.

In asampragyata samadhi there is a cessation of all
mental activity, and the mind only retains
unmanifested impressions.

Videhas and prakriti-layas attain asampragyata
samadhi because they ceased to identify themselves
with their bodies in their previous life.
They take rebirth because seeds of desire remained.

Others who attain asampragyata samadhi
attain through faith, effort, recollection, concentration,
and discrimination.

Patanjali is the greatest scientist of the inner; his approach is that of a scientific mind. He is not a poet. In that way he is very rare because those who enter the inner world are almost always poets; those who enter the outer world are almost always scientists.

He is a rare flower with a scientific mind, but his journey is inner. That's why he became the first and the last word: he is the alpha and the omega. In five thousand years nobody could improve upon him. And it seems he cannot be improved upon. He will remain the last word – because the very combination is impossible. It is almost impossible to have a scientific attitude and to enter the inner. He talks like a mathematician, a logician. He talks like Aristotle, and he is a Heraclitus.

Try to understand his every word. It will be difficult because his terms will be those of logic and reasoning, but his indication is toward love, ecstasy, godliness. His terminology is that of the man who works in a scientific lab, but his lab is one of the inner being. So don't be misguided by his terminology, just retain the feeling that he is a mathematician of the ultimate poetry. He is a paradox, but he never uses paradoxical language – he cannot. He retains a very firm logical background. He analyzes, dissects, but his aim is synthesis. He analyzes only to synthesize.

So always remember the goal: to reach to the ultimate through a scientific approach. And don't be misguided by the path. That's why Patanjali has impressed the Western mind so much. He has always been an influence. He has been an influence wherever his name has been heard because you can understand him easily – but to understand him is not enough. To understand him is as easy as to understand an Einstein. He talks to the intellect, but you have to remember this: his aim, his target, is the heart.

We will be moving on a dangerous terrain. If you forget that he is also a poet, you will be misguided. You will then become too attached to his terminology, language, reasoning, and forget his goal. He wants you to go through reasoning to go beyond it. That is a possibility. You can exhaust reasoning so deeply that you transcend it. You go through reasoning, you don't avoid it. You use reason as a step to go beyond. Now listen to his words. Each word has to be analyzed.

> Sampragyata samadhi is the samadhi that is
> accompanied by reasoning, reflection, bliss, and a
> sense of pure being.

He divides *samadhi*, the ultimate, into two steps. The ultimate cannot be divided. It is indivisible, in fact there are no steps. But just to help the mind, the seeker, he divides it first into two. The first step he calls *sampragyata samadhi* – a *samadhi* in which the mind is retained in its purity.

This first step: the mind has to be refined and purified – you cannot simply drop it. Patanjali says, "It is impossible to drop it because impurities have a tendency to cling. You can drop it only when the mind is absolutely pure – so refined, so subtle, that it has no tendency to cling."

He does not say, "Drop the mind," as Zen masters say. He says, "It is impossible to drop it. You are talking nonsense." You are saying the truth, but that's not possible because an impure mind has a weight – it hangs like a stone. And an impure mind has desires – millions of desires, unfulfilled, hankering to be fulfilled, asking to be fulfilled – with millions of incomplete thoughts in it. How can you drop it? The incomplete always tries to be completed. Patanjali says: "Remember, you can only drop a thing when it is complete."

Haven't you noticed? If you are an artist and painting a picture, unless you complete it, you cannot forget it. That picture continues to haunt you. You sleep badly; it is always there. There is an undercurrent in the mind. It moves, it asks to be completed. Once it is completed, it is finished. You can forget about it. The mind has a tendency toward completion. The mind is a perfectionist, so whatever is incomplete creates tension.

Patanjali says, "You cannot drop thinking unless it is so perfect that there is nothing more to be done; you can simply drop it and forget." This is diametrically opposite to Zen, to Heraclitus. The first *samadhi*, which is *samadhi* only for name's sake, is *sampragyata* – *samadhi* with a subtle purified mind. The second *samadhi* is *asampragyata* – *samadhi* with no mind. But Patanjali says, "When the mind disappears and there are no thoughts, then too subtle seeds of the past are retained by the unconscious."

The conscious mind is divided in two. First, *sampragyata* – the mind with a purified state, just like purified butter. It has a beauty of its own, but it is there. And however beautiful, the mind is ugly; however pure and silent, the very phenomenon of the mind is impure. You cannot purify a poison, it remains a poison. On the contrary, the more you purify it the more poisonous it becomes. It may look very, very beautiful; it may have its own color, shades, but it is still impure.

First you purify it, then you drop it. But still the journey is not complete because this is all in the conscious mind. What will you do with the unconscious mind? Just behind the layers of the conscious mind is a vast continent of the unconscious mind. In the unconscious are the seeds of all your past lives.

Patanjali divides the unconscious into two. He says, "*Sabeej samadhi*" – when the unconscious is there and the mind has been dropped consciously, it is a *samadhi* with seeds: *sabeej*. When those seeds are also burned, you attain the perfect – the *nirbeej samadhi*: *samadhi* without seeds.

So the conscious and the unconscious are in two steps. When *nirbeej samadhi*, the ultimate ecstasy, is reached… And without seeds within you to sprout and flower and to take you on further journeys into existence, you disappear.

In these sutras he says: *Sampragyata samadhi is the samadhi that is accompanied by reasoning, reflection, bliss, and a sense of pure being.* But this is the first step. Many are misguided; they think this is the last step because it is so pure. You feel so blissful and so happy that you think that now there is nothing more to be achieved. If you ask Patanjali, he will say, "The satori of Zen is just the first *samadhi*. It is not the final, the ultimate; the ultimate is still far away."

The words he uses cannot be exactly translated into English because Sanskrit is the most perfect language; no language comes even close to it. So I will have to explain it to you. The word used is *kutarka*. In English it is translated as reasoning. It is a poor translation. *Kutarka* has to be understood. *Tarka* means logic, reasoning. Patanjali says that there are three types of logic. One he calls *kutarka*: reasoning oriented toward the negative; always thinking in terms of no, denying, doubting, nihilistic.

Whatever you say to the man who lives in *kutarka* – negative logic – he always thinks how to deny it, how to say no to it. He looks to the negative. He is always complaining, grumbling. He always feels that something somewhere is wrong – always. You cannot put him right because this is his orientation. If you tell him to look at the sun, he will not see the sun, he will see the sunspots. He will always find the darker side of things; that is *kutarka*: wrong reasoning. But it looks like reasoning.

Finally, it leads to atheism. You deny God, because if you

cannot see the good, and the lighter side of life, how can you see God? You simply deny it. The whole of existence becomes dark. Everything is wrong, and you create a hell around you. If everything is wrong, how can you be happy? It is your creation, and you can always find something wrong because life consists of duality.

The rosebush has beautiful flowers, but also thorns. A man of *kutarka* will count the thorns, and come to an understanding that this rose must be illusory; it cannot exist. Amidst so many thorns, millions of thorns, how can a rose exist? It is impossible, the very possibility is denied. Somebody is deceiving you.

Mulla Nasruddin was feeling very, very sad. He went to the priest and said, "My crop is destroyed again – no rains. What can I do?"

The priest said, "Don't be so sad, Nasruddin. Look at the brighter side of life. You can be happy because you still have so much in your life. And always believe in God who is the provider. He even provides for the birds of the air, so why are you worried?"

Nasruddin replied, "Yes!" very bitterly. "Off my corn! God provides for the birds of the air off my corn."

He can't see the point. His crop is destroyed by the birds, and God is providing for them, "and my crop is destroyed." This type of mind always finds something or other, and is always tense. Anxiety will follow him like a shadow. This Patanjali calls *kutarka* – negative logic, negative reasoning.

Then there is *tarka* – simple reasoning. Simple reasoning leads nowhere. It moves in a circle because it has no goal. You can go on reasoning and reasoning, but you won't come to any conclusion because reasoning can come to a conclusion only when there is a goal at the very beginning. If you are moving in a direction, you reach somewhere. If you move in all directions – sometimes to the south, east, west – you waste energy.

Reasoning without a goal is called *tarka*. Reasoning with a negative attitude is called *kutarka*; reasoning with a positive grounding is called *vitarka*. *Vitarka* means special reasoning. So *vitarka* is the first element of *sampragyata samadhi*. A man who wants to attain inner peace has to be trained in *vitarka* – special reasoning. He always looks to the lighter side, the positive. He counts the flowers and forgets the thorns – not that there aren't any thorns, but he is not concerned with them. If you love the flowers and count them, a moment comes when you cannot believe in the thorns, because how can it be possible that thorns exist where there are so many beautiful flowers? It must be something illusory.

The man of *kutarka* counts the thorns, and the flowers become illusory. The man of *vitarka* counts the flowers, and the thorns become illusory. That's why Patanjali says, "*Vitarka* is the first element; only then is bliss possible. Through *vitarka* one attains heaven." One creates one's own heaven all around.

Your standpoint counts. Whatever you experience around you is your own creation – heaven or hell. Patanjali says, "You can go beyond logic and reasoning only through positive reasoning." You can never go beyond through the negative because the more you say no, the more you find things to be sad about, negative, denied. By and by, you have a constant no inside – a dark night with only thorns, and flowers unable to blossom in you, a desert.

When you say yes, you find more and more things to say yes to. When you say yes, you become a yea-sayer. Life is affirmed and you absorb all that is good and all that is true through your yes – beautiful. Yes becomes the door for the divine to enter you; no becomes a closed door. With your door closed, you are in hell; with all your doors open, existence flows in. You are fresh, young, alive; you become a flower.

Vitarka, vichar, ananda: Patanjali says, "If you are attuned with *vitarka* – a positive reasoning – you can be a thinker, but never before it. Only then does thinking arise." He has a very different meaning of thinking. You also think that you think; Patanjali will not agree. He says, "You have thoughts, but no thinking." That's why I say that it is difficult to translate him.

He says that you have thoughts, vagrant thoughts like a crowd, but no thinking. Between your two thoughts there is no inner current. They are uprooted things, there is no inner planning. Your thinking is a chaos, it is not a cosmos; it has no inner discipline. It is like when you look at a rosary: there are beads held together by an invisible thread running through them. Thoughts are beads; thinking is the thread. You have beads – too many, in fact, more than you need – but no inner running thread. Patanjali calls that inner thread thinking, *vichar*. You have thoughts, but no thinking. If this goes on and on, you will become mad. A madman is one who has millions of thoughts and no thinking. *Sampragyata samadhi* is the state when there are no thoughts, but thinking is perfect. This distinction has to be understood.

In the first place, your thoughts are not yours – you have gathered them together. Sometimes in a dark room, a beam of light comes from the roof and you can see millions of dust particles floating in that beam. When I look into you I see the same phenomenon: millions of dust particles. You call them thoughts. They are moving in you and out of you. From one head they enter another and on they go. They have their own life.

A thought is a thing; it has its own existence. When a person dies, all his mad thoughts are released immediately and they start finding shelter somewhere or other. They immediately enter those who are nearby. They are like germs, they have their own life. Even when you are alive you go on dispersing your thoughts all around you. When you talk, of course you throw your thoughts into others. But when you are silent, you also throw thoughts around. They are not yours; that is the first thing.

A man of positive reasoning will discard all thoughts that are not his own. They are not authentic, he hasn't found them through his own experience. He has accumulated them from others, they are borrowed. They are dirty, and have been in many hands and in many heads. A man of thinking does not borrow, he likes to have fresh thoughts of his own. If you are positive, and look at beauty, truth, goodness, flowers; if you become capable of seeing even in the darkest night that the morning is approaching – you will become capable of thinking.

You can then create your own thoughts. A thought that is created by you is really full of potential; it has a power of its own. These thoughts that you have borrowed are almost dead because they have been traveling – traveling for millions of years. Their origin is lost. They have lost all contact with their origin. They are just like dust floating around. You catch them – sometimes you even become aware of it, but because your awareness is such, it cannot see through things.

Sometimes you are sitting somewhere, and suddenly you become sad for no reason at all. You cannot find the reason why. You look around, you can find no reason; nothing is there, nothing has happened – you are just the same and suddenly a sadness takes over. A thought is passing; you are just in the way. It is an accident. A thought was passing like a cloud – a sad thought released by someone. It is an accident, and you are in the grip of it. Sometimes a thought persists – you don't see why you go on thinking about it. It looks absurd, it seems to be of no use. But you cannot do anything, it goes on knocking at the door. It says, "Think about me." A thought is waiting at the door, knocking. It says, "Give me some space. I would like to come in."

Each thought has its own life; it moves. It has such power and you are so impotent because you are so unaware that you are moved by thoughts. Your whole life consists of such accidents. You meet people, and your whole life pattern changes. Something enters in you, you are possessed, and you forget where you were going. You follow this thought, and change your direction. This is just an accident. You are like children.

Patanjali says, "This is not thinking. This is the state of absence of thinking; this is not thinking." You are a crowd. You haven't a center within you which can think. When one moves in the discipline of *vitarka*, right reasoning, by and by one becomes capable of thinking. Thinking is a capacity; thoughts are not. Thoughts can be learned from others; thinking, never. Thinking you have to learn yourself. This is the difference between the old Indian schools of learning and the modern universities. In modern universities you are receiving thoughts; in the ancient schools of learning – wisdom schools – they were teaching thinking, not thoughts.

Thinking is a quality of your inner being. What does thinking mean? – it means to retain your consciousness; to remain alert and aware, to encounter a problem. When a problem presents itself, you face it with your total awareness and an answer arises, a response. This is thinking.

A question is posed, you have a ready-made answer. Before you have even thought about it, the answer comes automatically. Someone says, "Is there a God?" He hasn't even uttered it before you say, "Yes." You nod your wooden head and say, "Yes, there is."

Is it your thought? Have you thought about the problem right this minute, or do you carry a ready-made answer in your memory? Someone gave it to you – your parents, teachers, society; someone has given it to you. You carry it as a precious treasure, and this answer comes from that memory.

A man of thinking uses his consciousness freshly each time there is a problem. He encounters the problem, and a thought arises within him which is not part of his memory. This is the difference. A man of thoughts is a man of memory; he has no thinking capacity. If you ask him a new question he will be at a loss, he cannot answer it. If you ask a question he knows the answer to, he will answer immediately. This is the difference between a pundit and a man who knows, a man who can think.

Patanjali says, "*Vitarka*, right reasoning, leads to reflection, *vichar, vichar,* reflection, leads to bliss." Of course, this is the first glimpse, and it is a glimpse; it will come and it will be lost. You cannot hold it for long. It is going to be just a glimpse. It's as if lightning happened for a moment and you saw all the darkness disappear – but the darkness returns again. It is as if the clouds disappeared and you saw the moon for a second – again the clouds return. Or, on a sunny morning near the Himalayas, you have a glimpse just for a moment of Gourishankar – the highest peak. But then there is mist and clouds, and the peak is lost. This is satori. That's why – never try to translate *satori* as *samadhi.* Satori is a glimpse. Much has to be done after it is attained. In fact, the real work starts after the first satori, the first glimpse, because then you have had a taste of the infinite. Now a real authentic search starts. Before it, it was just so-so, lukewarm, because you were not really confident, not certain of what you were doing, where you were going, what was happening.

Before it, it was a faith, a trust. Before it, a master was needed to show you, to bring you back again and again. After satori has happened, it is no longer a faith, it has become a knowing. Now the trust is not an effort; now you trust because your own experience has shown you. After the first glimpse, the real search starts. Before it, you are just going round and round. Right reasoning leads to right reflection, right reflection leads to a state of bliss, and this state of bliss leads to a sense of pure being.

A negative mind is always egoistic. And that is the impure state of being. You feel the "I," but you feel it for the wrong reasons. Just watch and you will see that the ego feeds on no. Whenever you say, "No," the ego arises. Whenever you say, "Yes," the ego cannot arise because it needs fight, challenge, to put itself against someone or something. It cannot exist alone, it needs duality. An egoist is always in search of a fight – with someone, with something, with some situation. He is always trying to find something to say no to – to win over, to be victorious.

The ego is violent, and no is the subtlest violence. When you say no to ordinary things, the ego arises even there. A small child says to its mother, "Can I go out to play?" and she says, "No" Nothing much was involved, but when the mother says no she feels she is someone. For instance you go to a railway station and ask for a ticket and the clerk simply doesn't look at you. He goes on working even if he has no work to do. But what he is saying is, "No, wait!" He feels he is someone, somebody. That's why, in offices everywhere you will hear, "No." Yes, is rare, very rare. An ordinary clerk can say no to anybody, whoever you are. He feels powerful. No gives you a sense of power – remember this. Unless it is absolutely necessary, never say no. Even if it is absolutely necessary, say it in such an affirmative way that the ego doesn't arise. You can say... Even no can be said in such a way that it appears like yes. You can say yes in such a way that it looks like no. It depends on the tone, the attitude, the gesture.

Remember this: for seekers, it has to be constantly remembered that you have to live continuously in the aroma of yes. That is what a man of faith is. He says, "Yes." Even when no is needed, he says, "Yes." He doesn't see that there is any antagonism in life. He affirms. He says yes to his body, his mind, and to everybody; he says yes to the total existence. The ultimate flowering happens when you can say a categorical yes, with no conditions. Suddenly the ego falls – it cannot stand up, it needs the props of no. The negative attitude creates the ego. With the positive attitude the ego drops, and the being is pure.

Sanskrit has two words for "I" – *ahankar* and *asmita*. It is difficult to translate. *Ahankar* is the wrong sense of "I" which comes from saying no. *Asmita* is the right sense of "I" which comes by saying yes. Both are "I." One is impure; no is the impurity – negate, destroy. No is destructive, a very subtle destruction. Never use it, drop it as often as you can. Whenever you are alert, don't use it. Even if you have to say it, try to find a roundabout way that has the appearance of yes. By and by you will become attuned, and you will feel through the yes such a purity coming to you.

And *asmita*; *asmita* is egoless ego. There is no feeling of "I" against anybody – just feeling oneself without putting yourself against anybody. Just feeling your total loneliness... And total loneliness is the purest of states. When we say "I am," "I" is *ahankar*, "am" is *asmita* – just the feeling of amness with no "I" to it, just feeling existence, the being. Yes is beautiful. No is ugly.

> In asampragyata samadhi there is a cessation of all
> mental activity, and the mind only retains
> unmanifested impressions.

Sampragyata samadhi is the first step: right reasoning, right reflection, a state of bliss, a glimpse of bliss, and a feeling of "amness." Pure simple existence without any ego in it – this leads to *asampragyata samadhi*. First is a purity, second is a disappearance because even the purest is impure because it is there. "I" is wrong; "am" is also wrong – better than "I," but a higher possibility is there when "am" also disappears – not only *ahankar*, but *asmita* too. You are impure, then you become pure, but if you start feeling, "I am pure," purity itself has become impurity. That too has to disappear.

The disappearance of purity is *asampragyata samadhi*; the disappearance of impurity is *sampragyata samadhi*. The disappearance of purity as well as impurity is *asampragyata*. There is a cessation of all mental activity. In the first state, thoughts disappear and in the second state, thinking also disappears. In the first state, thorns disappear; in the second state, flowers also disappear. When no disappears in the first state, yes remains. In the second state, yes also disappears because yes is also related to no. How can you retain yes without no? They are together, you cannot separate them. If no disappears, how can you say yes? Deep down yes is saying no to no. Negation of negation – but a subtle no exists. When you say yes, what are you doing? – you are not saying no, but the no is inside. You are not bringing it out; it is unmanifested.

THE MEANING OF SAMADHI

Your yes cannot mean anything if you haven't no within you. What will it mean? – it will be meaningless. Yes has meaning only because of no; no has meaning only because of yes. They are a duality.

In *sampragyata samadhi*, no is dropped; all that is wrong is dropped. In *asampragyata samadhi*, yes is dropped; all that is right, all that is good, that too is dropped. In *sampragyata samadhi* you drop the Devil; in *asampragyata samadhi* you also drop God, because how can God exist without the Devil? They are two aspects of the same coin.

All activity ceases. Yes is also an activity, and activity is a tension. Something is going on… Beautiful even, but still something is going on, and after a period even the beautiful becomes ugly. After a period of time you are bored with flowers; after a period of time, activity, even very subtle and pure, gives you tension; it becomes an anxiety. *In asampragyata samadhi there is a cessation of all mental activity, and the mind only retains unmanifested impressions.*

But still, it is not the goal. What will happen to all the impressions you have gathered in the past? For many, many lives you have lived, acted, reacted. You have done many things, undone many things. What will happen to it? The conscious mind has become pure; the conscious mind has dropped even the activity of purity. But the unconscious is vast and you carry all the seeds there, the blueprints. They are within you.

The tree has disappeared; you have cut down the tree completely – but the seeds that have fallen and are lying in the ground will sprout when their season comes. You will have another life, you will be born again. Of course, your quality will be different, but you will be born again because those seeds are yet to be burned.

You have cut down that which was manifested. It is easy to cut down anything that is in manifestation; it is easy to cut down all the trees. You can go into a garden and pull up all the grass on the lawn; you can kill everything, but within two weeks it will come up again because what you did was to pull up the manifested. You haven't touched the seeds which are lying in the soil. That has to be done in the third state.

Asampragyata samadhi is still *sabeej* – with seeds. And there are methods: how to burn those seeds, how to create fire – the fire that Heraclitus talked about – how to create that fire and burn the unconscious seeds. When they disappear, the soil is absolutely pure, and nothing can arise out of it. There is no birth, no death. The whole wheel stops for you, you have dropped out of the wheel. Dropping out of society won't help unless you drop out of the wheel. Then you become a perfect dropout!

Buddha is a perfect dropout; Mahavira, Patanjali, are perfect dropouts. They haven't only dropped out of the establishment or society, they have dropped out of the very wheel of life and death. But that happens only when all the seeds are burned. The final is *nirbeej samadhi* – seedless.

> In asampragyata samadhi there is a cessation of all
> mental activity, and the mind only retains
> unmanifested impressions.

> Videhas and prakriti-layas attain asampragyata
> samadhi because they ceased to identify themselves
> with their bodies in their previous life.
> They take rebirth because seeds of desire remained.

Even a Buddha is born if in his past life he attained *asampragyata samadhi*, but the seeds were there. He had to come once more. Even a Mahavira is born – once; the seeds bring him. But this is going to be the last life. After *asampragyata samadhi*, only one life is possible. But the quality of this life will be totally different because this man will not be identified with the body. This man really has nothing to do because the activity of the mind has ceased. What will he do? And why is this one life

THE MEANING OF SAMADHI

needed? He has just to allow those seeds to be manifested and he will remain a witness. This is the fire.

A man came to Buddha and spat on him; the man was very angry. Buddha wiped his face and asked, "What else do you have to say?"

The man couldn't understand it, he was really angry – red-hot. He couldn't even understand what Buddha was saying. The whole thing was so absurd because Buddha didn't react. The man was at a loss – what to do, what to say. He went away, and couldn't sleep the whole night. How can you sleep when you insult somebody and there is no reaction? Your insult comes back to you. You threw the arrow; it has not been received. It comes back. Finding no shelter, it comes back to the source. He insulted Buddha, but the insult couldn't find a shelter there, so where will it go? – it comes back to the original master.

The whole night he was feverish; he couldn't believe what had happened. He started repenting – that he was wrong, that he had not done a good thing. Early next morning he went and asked for forgiveness.

Buddha said, "Don't worry about it. I must have done something wrong to you in the past. Now the account is closed. I am not going to react; otherwise again and again... Finished! I have not reacted because it was a seed somewhere and it had to be finished. Now my account with you is closed."

In this life, when a *videha* – one who has understood that he is not the body, who has attained *asampragyata samadhi* – comes in the world, it is just to finish accounts. His whole life consists of finishing accounts; millions of lives, many relationships, many involvements, commitments – everything has to be closed.

It happened...

Buddha arrived at a village; the whole village had gathered

17

THE HEART OF YOGA

together, and they were eager to listen to him. It was a rare opportunity because even the capital cities were continually inviting him, and he never visited. He had come to this small, out-of-the-way village without any invitation. The villagers would never have gathered enough courage to ask him to come to their village. It was small with just a few huts, and he had arrived without an invitation! The whole village was afire with excitement, and he was sitting under a tree and not speaking.

They asked him, "Who are you waiting for? Everybody is here; the whole village is here. You can start."

Buddha replied, "But I have to wait because I have come for someone who is not here. A promise has to be fulfilled, an account closed. I am waiting for that one."

A girl arrived, and Buddha started. After he had finished speaking, they asked him, "Were you waiting for this girl?" The girl belonged to the untouchables, to the lowest caste. Nobody thought that Buddha was waiting for her.

He replied, "Yes, I was waiting for her. When I was traveling here, she met me on the road and said, 'Wait, because I am going to the other town for some work, but I will come soon.' Somewhere in a past life I had given her a promise that when I became enlightened I would come and tell her what had happened to me. That account has to be closed. That promise is hanging on to me and if I cannot fulfill it, I will have to come again."

A *videha* or a *prakriti-laya*… Both words are beautiful. *Videha* means bodiless. When you attain *asampragyata samadhi* the body is present, but you become bodiless. You are no longer the body. The body becomes the abode – you are not identified with it.

So these two terms are beautiful. *Videha* means one who knows that he is not the body – he knows, remember, not believes. And *prakriti-laya*, because one who knows that he is not the body, is no longer the *prakriti*, the nature.

The body belongs to the material. Once you're not identified with the matter within you, you are not identified with the matter without, outside. A man who attains the state that he is no longer a body, attains that he is no longer the manifested, the *prakriti* – his nature is dissolved. There is no longer "the world" for him; he is not identified, he has become a witness to it. Such a man is also born at least once because he has to close many accounts; many promises have to be fulfilled, many karmas to be dropped.

It happened...

Buddha's cousin, Devadatta, was against him; he tried to kill him in many different ways. Once, when Buddha was sitting under a tree, meditating, Devadatta pushed a big rock down from the top of a hill. Everyone ran away as the rock rolled down. Buddha remained there sitting under the tree – it was dangerous, the rock rolled down just touching him, brushing him.

Ananda asked him, "Why didn't you get out of the way when we all did? There was enough time."

Buddha replied, "There is enough time for you. My time is over. Devadatta has to do it. In the past, in some other life there was some karma. I must have given him some pain, some anguish, some anxiety. It has to be closed. If I escape, if I do anything, a new line starts again."

A *videha*, a man who has attained *asampragyata*, does not react. He simply watches, witnesses. This is the fire of witnessing which burns all the seeds in the unconscious, and a moment comes when the soil is absolutely pure; there is no seed waiting to sprout. Then there is no need to come back. First the nature dissolves, and then he dissolves himself into the universe.

Videhas and prakriti-layas attain asampragyata samadhi because they ceased to identify themselves with their bodies in their previous life. They take rebirth because seeds of desire remained. I am here to fulfill something; you are here to close my account. You are not here accidentally. There are millions of people in the world. Why are you here and not somebody else? Something has to be closed.

Others who attain asampragyata samadhi attain
through faith, effort, recollection, concentration, and
discrimination.

So these are the two possibilities. If you have attained *asampragyata samadhi* in your past life, in this life you are born a buddha – just a few seeds have to be fulfilled, have to be dropped, burned. That's why I say that you are born almost a buddha. There is no need for you to do anything, you simply have to watch whatever happens.

Hence Krishnamurti's continuous insistence that there is no need to do anything. It is right for him, it is not right for his listeners. For his listeners, there is much that needs to be done, and they will be misguided by this statement. He is speaking about himself. He was born an *asampragyata* buddha, he was born a *videha*, he was born a *prakriti-laya*.

When he was just five years old he was taking a bath near Adyar, and one of the greatest Theosophists, Leadbeater, was watching him. He was a totally different type of child. If somebody threw mud at him, he would not react. There were many children playing there. If somebody pushed him into the river, he would simply go with it. Yes, he was not angry, he was not fighting. He had a totally different quality – the quality of an *asampragyata* buddha.

Leadbeater called Annie Besant and told her to watch this child. He was no ordinary child, and the whole Theosophical movement whirled around him. They hoped very much that he would become an avatar – that he would become the perfect master for this age. But the problem was very deep.

They had chosen the right person, but they hoped wrongly – because a man who is born an *asampragyata* buddha cannot even be active as an avatar. All activity has ceased. He can simply watch – he can be a witness. You cannot make him very active.

He can be only a passivity. They had chosen the right person, but still wrong...

They hoped very much... And the whole movement whirled around Krishnamurti. When he dropped out and said, "I cannot do anything because nothing is needed," the whole movement flopped because they had too many hopes for him, and the whole thing turned out completely differently. But this could have been prophesied.

Annie Besant, Leadbeater and others, were very beautiful people, but not really aware of Eastern methods. They had learned a lot from books, scriptures, but they did not exactly know the secret which Patanjali is showing: that an *asampragyata*, a *videha*, is born, but he is not active. He is a passivity. So much can happen through him, but that can happen only if somebody comes and surrenders to him. He is a passivity, he cannot force you to do something. He is available, but he cannot be aggressive.

His invitation is for everybody and for all. It is an open invitation, but he cannot send you a particular invitation because he cannot be active. He is an open door; if you like, you can pass through. The last life is an absolute passivity, just witnessing. This is one way *asampragyata* buddhas are born from their past life.

But you can become an *asampragyata* buddha in this life too. For them Patanjali says, "*Shraddha virya smriti samadhi pragya.*" *Others who attain asampragyata samadhi attain through faith, effort, recollection, concentration, and discrimination.* It is almost impossible to translate it, so I will explain rather than translate – just to give you the feel, because the words will misguide you.

Shraddha is not exactly faith, it is more like trust. Trust is very, very different from faith. Faith is something you are born into, trust is something you grow in. Hinduism is a faith; to be a Christian is a faith, to be a Mohammedan is a faith. But to be a disciple here with me is a trust. Remember – I cannot claim faith. Jesus also could not claim faith because faith is something you are born into. Jews were faithful; they had faith. In fact, that is why they destroyed Jesus because they thought that he was bringing them out of their faith, and destroying it. He was asking for trust. Trust is a personal intimacy, it is not a social phenomenon. You attain it through your own response. Nobody can be born in trust; in faith, okay.

Faith is dead trust, trust is alive faith.

So try to understand the distinction. One has to grow in *shraddha*, trust – it is always personal. The first disciples of Jesus attained trust. They were Jews, born Jews. They moved out of their faith. It is a rebellion.

Faith is a superstition; trust is a rebellion.

First, trust leads you away from your faith. It has to be so because if you are living in a dead graveyard, first you have to be led out of it. Only then can you be introduced to life again. Jesus was trying to bring people toward *shraddha*, trust. It will always look as if he is destroying their faith.

Now when a Christian comes to me, the same situation is repeated. Christianity is a faith, just as Judaism was a faith in Jesus' time. When a Christian comes to me, once again I have to bring him out of his faith to help him grow toward trust. Religions are faith, and to be religious is to be in trust. To be religious doesn't mean to be Christian, Hindu, or Mohammedan because trust has no name; it is not labeled. It is like love. Is love Christian, Hindu, Mohammedan? Is marriage Christian, Hindu, Mohammedan? Love? Love knows no caste, no distinctions. Love doesn't know if you are a Hindu or a Christian.

Marriage is like faith; love is like trust – you have to grow into it, it is an adventure. Faith is not an adventure; you are born into it, it is convenient. If you are seeking comfort and convenience, it is better to remain in faith. Be a Hindu, a Christian; follow the rules. But it will remain a dead thing unless you respond from your heart, unless you enter religion on your own responsibility, and not because you were born a Christian. How can you be born a Christian?

How is religion associated with birth? Birth cannot give you religion. It can give you a society, a creed, a sect; it can give you a superstition. The word *superstition* is very, very meaningful. It means, unnecessary faith. The word *super* means unnecessary, superfluous – faith which has become unnecessary, faith which has died. At some time it may have been alive.

Religion has to be reborn again and again. Remember, you are not born in a religion. Religion has to be born in you, then it is trust – again and again. You cannot give your children your religion, they will have to seek and find their own. Everybody has to seek and find his own. It is an adventure – the greatest adventure. You move into the unknown.

Patanjali says that if you want to attain *asampragyata samadhi*, *shraddha* is the first thing. And for *sampragyata samadhi*, reasoning, right reasoning. See the distinction? – for *sampragyata samadhi*, right reasoning, right thinking is the base; for *asampragyata samadhi*, right trust – not reasoning.

No reasoning… But a love. And love is blind. It looks blind to reason because it is a jump into the dark. Reason asks, "Where are you going? Remain in the known territory. What is the use of moving to a new phenomenon? Why not remain in the old fold? It is convenient, comfortable, and whatever you need, it can supply." But everybody has to find his own temple. Only then is it alive.

You are here with me – this is trust. When I am no longer here, your children may be with me. That will be faith. Trust happens only with a living master, faith happens with dead masters who are no longer there. The first disciples have the religion.

By and by, the second and third generation loses the religion, it becomes a sect. You simply follow because you are born into it. It is a duty, not a love. It is a social code. It helps, but it hasn't gone deep in you. It brings nothing to you; it is not a happening. It is not a depth unfolding in you – it is just a surface, a face. Just go and look in the church: the Sunday people attend, they even pray. But they are just waiting for it to finish.

A small child was sitting in church. He was just four years old and had come for the first time. His mother asked him how he liked it.

He replied, "The music is good, but the commercial is too long."

It is a commercial when you have no trust. *Shraddha* is right trust; faith is wrong trust. Don't take religion from somebody else. You cannot borrow it; that is a deception. You are getting it without paying for it, and everything has to be paid for. And to attain *asampragyata samadhi* is not cheap. You have to pay the full cost, and the full cost is your total being.

To be a Christian is just a label. To be religious is not a label, your whole being is involved. It is a commitment. Some people come to me and say, "We love you. Whatever you say is good. But we don't want to take sannyas because we don't want to commit ourselves." But unless you are committed, involved, you cannot grow, because there is no relationship. There are just words between you and me, not a relationship. I may be a teacher to you, but not a master. You may be a student, but not a disciple.

The first door is *shraddha*, trust; the second is *virya*. That too is difficult. It is translated as *effort*. No, effort is simply a part of it. The word *virya* means many things, but deep down it means bioenergy. One of the meanings of *virya* is semen, sexual potency. If you really want to translate it exactly, *virya* is bioenergy, your total energy phenomenon – you as energy. Of course, this energy can be brought only through effort; hence, one of the meanings is *effort*.

But that is poor – not as rich as the word *virya*. *Virya* means that your total energy has to be brought into it. With only the mind, it won't do. You can say yes from the mind, but that will not be enough. That is the meaning of *virya*: your totality, without holding anything back. And that is possible only when there is trust. Otherwise you will hold on to something, just to be secure and safe because who knows, "This man may be leading us in the wrong direction, so we can step back at any moment. Any moment we can say, 'Enough is enough; now no more.'"

You hold back a part of you just to be watchful. Where is this man leading us? People come to me and say, "We are just watching. First let us watch what is happening." They are very clever – clever fools because these things cannot be watched from the outside. What is happening is an inner phenomenon. Many times you cannot even see to whom it is happening. Many times only I can see what is happening. Only later on do you become aware of what has happened.

Others cannot watch. There is no possibility of watching it from the outside. How can you watch from the outside? You can see gestures; you can see people doing meditation, but what is happening inside, that is meditation. What they are doing outside is just creating a situation.

It happened…

There was a great Sufi master, Jalaluddin. He had a small school of rare pupils – rare, because he was a very choosy master. He would not accept anyone unless he had chosen the person himself. He worked with very few, but sometimes people passing by would come to see what was happening there.

Once, a group of professors came to his school. Always being very alert, clever people, they decided to have a look for themselves. In the master's house, which was in the compound, a group of fifty people were sitting, making mad gestures – someone was laughing, someone was crying, someone was jumping around. The professors watched and said, "What's going on? This man is leading these people into madness. They are already mad, and are fools. And once you become mad it's difficult to come back. This is nonsense; we have never heard of… People sit silently when they meditate."

There was a lot of discussion between them. Eventually, a group of them said, "We don't know what is happening, so it's better not to make any judgment."

There was a third group among them who said, "Whatever it is, it is worth enjoying. We would like to watch. It looks beautiful. Why can't we enjoy it? Why be bothered about what they are doing? Just to watch is a beautiful thing."

After a few months, the same group of professors came again to the school to watch. What was happening now? – everyone was silent. Again there were fifty people, and the master was also there. They were sitting silently, so silently, as if there was no one there, like statues. Again they had a discussion. One group said, "Now they are useless. There is nothing to see! When we came the first time it was beautiful. We enjoyed it. But now they are just boring."

The other group said, "But now we think they are meditating. The first time they were simply mad. This is the right thing to do, this is how meditation is done. It is written in the scriptures and described in this way."

But there was still a third group who said, "We don't know anything about meditation. How can we judge?"

After a few months, the group came again. Now there was nobody there. Only the master was sitting, smiling. All the disciples had disappeared. They asked, "What is happening? The first time we came there was a mad crowd here and we thought that this is useless, you are driving people crazy. The next time we came it was very good. People were meditating. Where have they all gone?"

The master replied, "The work is done, the disciples have disappeared. I am happily smiling because the thing happened. And I know that you are the fools! I have also been watching – not only you. I know what discussions were going on between you, and what you were thinking the first and second time you came." Jalaluddin continued, "The effort that you have made in coming

here three times would have been enough for you to become med-
itators, and the discussion that you have been involved in, that
much energy was enough to make you silent. In the same period,
those disciples have disappeared and you are standing at the same
place. Come in! Don't watch from the outside."

They said, "Yes, that is why we came again and again, to watch
what was happening. When we are certain, okay. Otherwise we
don't want to be committed."

Clever people never want to commit, but is there life without
commitment? Clever people think commitment is a bondage, but
is there any freedom without bondage? First you have to move
into a relationship, only then can you go beyond it. First, you
have to move into a deep commitment, depth to depth, heart to
heart. Only then can you transcend it. There is no other way. If
you just move out and watch, you can never enter the shrine. And
there can be no relationship. The shrine is commitment.

A master and disciple is a love relationship, the highest love
that is possible. And unless there is a relationship you cannot
grow. Patanjali says: "The first is trust – *shraddha*; the second is
energy – effort." You have to bring your whole energy in; a part
won't do. It may even be destructive if you only come partially
in and remain partially out because that will become a rift within
you. It will create a tension within you; it will become an anxiety
rather than bliss.

Bliss is where you are in your totality; anxiety is where you
are only in part because you are divided and there is a tension.
The two parts are going separate ways. You are in difficulty.

*Others who attain asampragyata samadhi attain through
faith...* trust, effort, energy, recollection. This word *recollection*
is *smriti*: remembrance – what Gurdjieff calls self-remembering.
That is *smriti*.

You don't remember yourself. You may remember millions
of things but you go on continuously forgetting yourself – that

you are. Gurdjieff had a technique; he got it from Patanjali. In fact, all techniques come from Patanjali. He is the past master of techniques. *Smriti* is remembrance – self-remembering, whatever you do. You are walking; remember deep down, "I am walking, I am." Don't be lost in walking. Walking is happening – the movement, the activity – and the inner center is there, just aware, watching, witnessing. You need not repeat it in the mind, "I am walking." If you repeat it, that is not remembrance. You have to be nonverbally aware: "I am walking, I am eating, I am talking, I am listening." Whatever you do, the "I" inside should not be forgotten, it should remain. It is not self-consciousness, it is consciousness of the self. Self-consciousness is ego; consciousness of the self is *asmita*, purity, just being aware that "I am."

Ordinarily, your consciousness is arrowed toward an object. You look at me, and your whole consciousness is moving toward me like an arrow. But you are arrowed toward me. Self-remembering means you must have a double-arrowed arrow, one side showing me, another side showing you. A double-arrowed arrow is *smriti*, self-remembrance – very difficult because it is easy to remember the object and forget yourself. The opposite is also easy – to remember yourself and forget the object. Both are easy; that's why those who are in the market, in the world, and those who are in the monastery, out of the world, are the same. Both are single-arrowed. In the market they are looking at things, objects. In the monastery they are looking at themselves.

Smriti is neither in the market nor in the monastery. *Smriti* is a phenomenon of self-remembering, when subject and object are both together in consciousness. That is the most difficult thing in the world. Even if you attain for a single moment, a split moment, you will have the glimpse of satori immediately. Immediately you have moved out of the body... Somewhere else.

Try it. But, remember, if you don't have trust it will become a tension. These are the problems involved. It will become such a tension that you could go mad because it is a very tense state.

That's why it is difficult to remember both: the object and the subject, the outer and the inner. To remember both is very, very arduous. If there is trust, that trust will decrease the tension – because trust is love. It will soothe you; it will be a soothing force around you. Otherwise the tension can become so much that you will not be able to sleep. You will not be at peace for one moment because it will be a constant problem, and you will be continuously anxious.

That's why we can do just one: go to the monastery, close your eyes, remember yourself, forget the world – that's easy. But what are you doing? – you have simply reversed the whole process, nothing else. No change. Or, forget the monasteries, the temples, the masters and be in the world, enjoy the world. That too is easy. The difficult thing is to be conscious of both. When you are conscious of both and the energy is simultaneously aware, arrowed in the diametrically opposite, there is transcendence. You simply become the third; you become the witness of both. When the third enters, you first try to see the object and yourself. But if you try to see both, by and by, you will feel something is happening within you – because you are becoming a third; you are between the two, the object and the subject. You are neither the object nor the subject now. ...*attain through faith, effort, recollection, concentration, and discrimination.*

Shraddha – trust, and *virya* – total commitment, effort, energy have to be brought in; all your potentiality has to be brought in. If you are really a seeker of truth you cannot seek anything else. It is a complete involvement. You cannot make it a part-time job: "Sometimes in the morning I meditate and then I go out." No, meditation has to become a twenty-four-hour continuity. Whatever you do, meditation has to be continuously there in the background. Energy will be needed; your whole energy will be needed.

And now, a few things: if your whole energy is needed, sex disappears automatically because you don't have energy to waste.

Brahmacharya for Patanjali is not a discipline, it is a conse-quence. You put your total energy in, so you don't have any energy left. It happens in ordinary life too. Watch a great painter; he forgets women completely. When he is painting there is no sex in his mind because his whole energy is moving. You don't have any extra energy.

A great poet, a great singer, a dancer who is moving totally in his commitment, automatically becomes celibate. He has no disci-pline for it. Sex is superfluous energy; it is a safety valve. When you have too much in you and you cannot do anything with it, nature has made a safety valve. You can throw it out, you can release it; otherwise you will go mad or burst, explode. If you try to suppress it, then too you will go mad because suppressing it won't help. It needs a transformation, and that transformation comes from total commitment. A warrior, if he is really a warrior, an impeccable warrior, will be beyond sex. His whole energy is moving.

A very, very beautiful story is reported...

There was a great philosopher, thinker. His name was Vachaspati. He was so involved in his studies that when his father said to him, "Now I am getting old, I don't know when I will die, maybe any moment, and you are my only son. I would like you to be married," he was so involved in his studies that he said, "Okay." He didn't hear what his father was saying. So he married. He married, but completely forgot that he had a wife because he was so involved.

This can happen only in India; this cannot happen anywhere else. His wife loved him so much that she never wanted to disturb him. So, it is said that twelve years passed. She served him like a shadow, taking every care, but without disturbing or saying, "I am here. What are you doing?" He was continuously writing a com-mentary – one of the greatest ever written. He was writing a commentary on Badarayana's *Brahma Sutra,* and he was so involved, so total, that he not only forgot about his wife, he was not even aware who had brought the food, who had taken the plates back, who came in the evening and lit the lamp, who had prepared his bed.

Twelve years passed, and the night arrived when his commentary was complete. He only had to write the last word, and he had taken a vow that when the commentary was complete, he would become a sannyasin. Then he would not be concerned with the mind, and everything would be finished. This was his only karma that had to be fulfilled.

That night he was a little more relaxed because he had written the last sentence nearabout twelve o'clock, and for the first time he became aware of his surroundings. The lamp was burning low and needed more oil. A beautiful hand was pouring oil into it. He looked again to see who was there. He didn't recognize the face. He said, "Who are you and what are you doing here?"

His wife replied, "Now that you have asked, I must tell you that twelve years ago you brought me here as your wife, but you were so involved, so committed to your work, that I didn't like to interrupt or disturb you."

Vachaspati started weeping, his tears started flowing. The wife asked, "What is the matter?"

He replied, "This is very complex. Now I am at a loss because the commentary is complete and I am a sannyasin. I cannot be a householder, I cannot be your husband. The commentary is complete, and I had taken a vow and now there is no time left for me here, I am going to leave immediately. Why didn't you tell me before? I could have loved you. What can I do for all your service, your love, your devotion?"

So he called his commentary on the *Brahma Sutra*, *Bhamati*. Bhamati was the name of his wife. The name is absurd – to call Badarayana's *Brahma Sutra* commentary, *Bhamati*... It has no relationship. He continued, "Now I can't do anything else. The last thing to do is to write the title of the book, so I will call it *Bhamati*, so that it is always remembered."

He left the house. His wife was weeping, crying – not in pain, but in absolute bliss. She said, "That's enough. This gesture, this love in your eyes, is enough. I have received enough; don't feel guilty. Go! And forget me completely. I wouldn't like to be a burden on your mind. There is no need to remember me."

It is possible… If you are totally involved, sex disappears because sex is a safety valve. When you have unused energy, sex becomes a thing haunting you all around. When your total energy is used, sex disappears. That is the state of *brahmacharya*, of *virya*, of all your potential energy flowering: *…effort, recollection, concentration, and discrimination.*

Shraddha – trust; *virya* – your total bioenergy, your total commitment and effort; *smriti* – self-remembrance. And *samadhi*. The word *samadhi* means a state of mind where no problem exists. It comes from the word *samadhan* – a state of mind when you feel absolutely okay, no problem, no question, a nonquestioning, nonproblematic state of mind. It is not concentration. Concentration is just a quality that comes to the mind that is without problems. This is the difficulty in translating. Concentration is part – it happens. Look at a child who is absorbed in play; he has a concentration without any effort. He is not concentrating on his play; concentration is a by-product. He is so absorbed in the play that concentration happens. If you knowingly concentrate on something, there is effort, there is tension, and you will be tired.

If you are absorbed, *samadhi* happens automatically, spontaneously. If you are listening to me, it is a *samadh*i. If you listen to me totally, there is no need for any other meditation. It becomes a concentration. It is not that you concentrate – if you listen lovingly, concentration follows.

In *asampragyata samadhi*, when trust is complete, when effort is total, when remembrance is deep, *samadhi* happens. Whatever you do, you do with total concentration – without any effort to *do* concentration. If concentration needs effort, it is ugly. It will be like a disease in you, you will be destroyed by it. Concentration should be a consequence. You love a person, and just being with him you are concentrated. Remember never to concentrate on anything. Rather listen deeply, listen totally, and concentration will come by itself.

And discrimination – *pragya*. *Pragya* is not discrimination; discrimination is again a part of *pragya*. In fact, *pragya* means wisdom – a knowing awareness. Buddha has said, "When the flame of meditation burns high, the light that surrounds that flame is *pragya*." *Samadhi* inside, and a light all around, an aura follows you. You are wise in your every act; not that you are trying to be wise, it simply happens because you are so totally aware. Whatever you do, it happens to be wise – not that you are continuously thinking about doing the right thing. A man who is continuously thinking about doing the right thing will not be able to do anything – he will not be able to do even the wrong thing because this will become such a tension on his mind.

How can you decide what is right and what is wrong? A man of wisdom, a man of understanding, does not choose. He simply feels. He simply throws his awareness everywhere, and in that light he moves. Wherever he moves is right.

Right does not belong to things, it belongs to you – the one who is moving. It is not that Buddha did right things – no. Whatever he did was right. *Discrimination* is a poor word. A man of understanding has discrimination. He doesn't think about it, it is just easy for him. If you want to get out of this room, you simply walk out the door. You don't grope, you don't go to the wall first and try to find the way, you simply go out. You don't even think that this is the door.

But when a blind man needs to go out, he asks, "Where is the door?" He also tries to find it. He knocks on various places with his cane, he will grope, and in his mind he goes on thinking, "Is this the door or the wall? Am I going the right way or the wrong way?" And when he comes to the door, he thinks, "Yes, now this is the door." All this happens because he is blind.

You have to discriminate because you are blind; you have to think because you are blind; you have to believe in right and wrong because you are blind; you have to be involved in discipline and morality because you are blind. When understanding flowers, and the flame is there, you simply see and everything is clear. When you have an inner clarity, everything is clear; you become perceptive. Whatever you do is simply right. Not that it is right, so you do it; you do it with understanding, and it is right.

Shraddha, virya, smriti, samadhi, pragya. Others who attain *asampragyata samadhi* attain through trust, infinite energy, effort, total self-remembrance, a nonquestioning mind and a flame of understanding.

Enough for today.

2

Simplicity Never Appeals
to the Ego

The first question:

Osho,
What you have been saying about Heraclitus, Christ,
and Zen seems like kindergarten teachings compared
to Patanjali. Heraclitus, Christ, and Zen make the final
step seem close; Patanjali makes even the first step
seem almost impossible. It seems like we Westerners
have hardly begun to realize the amount of work that
has to be done.

Lao Tzu says, "If Tao were not laughed at, it would not be Tao."
And I would like to say to you: "If you did not misunderstand me,
you would not be you. You are bound to misunderstand." You have
not understood what I had been saying about Heraclitus, Christ,
and Zen. If you cannot understand Heraclitus, Zen, and Jesus, you
will not be able to understand Patanjali either.

The first rule of understanding is not to compare. How can
you compare? What do you know about the innermost state of
Heraclitus, Basho, Buddha, Jesus or Patanjali? Who are you to
compare? Comparison is a judgment. Who are you to judge?
But the mind wants to judge because in judging the mind feels

superior. You become the judge and your ego feels very, very good. You feed the ego. Through judgment and comparison you think that you know.

They are different types of flowers – incomparable. How can you compare a rose with a lotus? Is any comparison possible? There's no possibility because both are different worlds. How can you compare the moon with the sun? There is no possibility because they are different dimensions. Heraclitus is a wildflower; Patanjali is in a cultivated garden. Patanjali will be nearer your intellect, Heraclitus nearer your heart. But as you go deeper, the differences are lost. When you start flowering, a new understanding dawns upon you – the understanding that flowers differ in their color, smell, shape, form and name.

But in flowering they don't differ. The flowering, the phenomenon that they have flowered, is the same. Heraclitus is, of course, different; he has to be. Every individual is unique. Patanjali is also different. You cannot put them into one category. No pigeonholes exist where you can force them or categorize them. But if you also flower, you will come to understand that flowering is the same whether the flower is a lotus or a rose. It makes no difference. The innermost phenomenon of energy coming to a celebration is the same.

Patanjali is a scientific thinker. He is a grammarian, a linguist. Heraclitus is a wild poet. They talk differently, they have different mind patterns. Heraclitus does not bother about grammar, language or form. When you say that listening to Patanjali you feel that Heraclitus, Basho, and Zen appear childish, like kindergarten teachings, you are not saying anything about Patanjali or Heraclitus, you are saying something about yourself. You are saying that you are a mind oriented person.

You can understand Patanjali; Heraclitus simply eludes you. Patanjali is more solid, you can have a grip on him. Heraclitus is a cloud, you cannot have any grip on him. You can make head and tail out of Patanjali, he seems rational. What will you do

with a Heraclitus, with a Basho? No, they are simply so irrational. Thinking about them, your mind becomes absolutely
impotent. When you say such things and make comparisons,
judgments, you say something about yourself – who you are.

Patanjali can be understood, there is no trouble about it. He
is absolutely rational and can be followed; there is no problem
there. All his techniques can be done because he gives you "the
how," and "how" is always easy to understand. What to do?
How to do it? He gives you the techniques.

Ask Basho or Heraclitus what to do, and they simply say,
"There is nothing to be done." You are at a loss. If something is
to be done you can do it, but if nothing is to be done you are at a
loss. Still, you go on asking again and again, "What to do? How
to do it? How to achieve that which you are talking about?"

They talk about the ultimate without talking about the way
that leads to it. Patanjali talks about the way, never about the
goal. He is concerned with the means, Heraclitus with the end.
The end is mysterious. It is poetry; it is not a mathematical solu-
tion. It is a mystery. But the path is a scientific thing. The
technique, the know-how appeals to you. But this shows something about you, not about Heraclitus or Patanjali. You are a
mind oriented person, a head oriented person. Try to see this.
Don't compare Patanjali and Heraclitus. Simply try to see that it
shows something about you. And if it shows something about
you, you can do something about it.

Don't think that you know what Patanjali is and what
Heraclitus is. You can't even understand an ordinary flower in
the garden – and they are the ultimate flowering in existence.
Unless you flower in the same way, you will not be able to
understand. But you can compare, you can judge, and through
judgment you will miss the whole point.

So the first rule of understanding is never to judge. Never
judge and never compare Buddha, Mahavira, Mohammed,
Christ, Krishna. Never compare! They exist in a dimension

beyond comparison, and whatever you know about them is really nothing – just fragments. You cannot have the total comprehension. They are so beyond. In fact, you simply see their reflection in the water of your mind.

You have not seen the moon; you have seen the moon in the lake. You have not seen the reality; you have simply seen a mirror reflection, and the reflection depends on the mirror. If the mirror is defective, the reflection is different. Your mind is your mirror.

When you say that Patanjali and his teaching seems very great, you are simply saying that you couldn't understand Heraclitus at all. If you cannot understand him, that simply shows that he is very, very far beyond you; he is further beyond you than Patanjali is. At least you can understand this much: that Patanjali seems to be difficult. Now follow me closely and if something is difficult, you can tackle it – however difficult, you can tackle it. More hard effort is needed, but that can be done.

Heraclitus is not easy, he is simply impossible. Patanjali is difficult. You can understand the difficult; you can do something. You can bring your will, effort, and your whole energy to it and it can be solved. The difficult can be made easy, and more subtle methods can be found. But what will you do with the impossible? It cannot be made easy, but you can deceive yourself. You can say that there is nothing in it, that it is a kindergarten teaching and you are so grown-up, that it is for children, not for you.

This is a trick of the mind to avoid the impossible because you know that you will not be able to tackle it. So the easiest course is simply to say, "It is not for me, it is below me – a kindergarten teaching." And you are a grown-up mature person. You need a university, you don't need a kindergarten. Patanjali suits you. He looks very difficult, but he can be solved. The impossible cannot be solved.

If you want to understand Heraclitus, there is no way except by dropping your mind completely. If you want to understand

THE HEART OF YOGA

Patanjali, there is a gradual way. He gives you steps – what to do – but remember, finally, eventually, he will also say to you, "Drop the mind." What Heraclitus says in the beginning, he will say in the end. But you can be fooled the whole way on the path. In the end he is going to say the same thing, but he will still be understandable because he makes grades; the jump doesn't look like a jump when you have steps.

This is the situation: Heraclitus just brings you to an abyss and says, "Jump!" You look down, your mind simply cannot comprehend what he is saying. It looks suicidal. There are no steps. You ask, "How?" and he says, "There is no 'how,' you simply jump!" What is the "how"? And because there are no steps, "how" cannot be explained. You simply jump! He says, "If you are ready I can push you, but there are no methods." Is there any method in taking a jump? A jump is sudden; methods exist when a thing, a process is gradual. Finding it impossible, you make an about-turn. To console yourself that you are not such a weakling you say that it is for children – it is not difficult enough. It is not for you.

Patanjali brings you to the same abyss, but he has made steps. He says, "Take one step at a time." It appeals – you can understand it. The mathematics is simple: take one step, then another. There is no jump. But remember, sooner or later he will bring you to the point from where you have to jump. He has created steps, but they don't lead to the bottom, just to the middle – and the bottom is so far away that you can exactly say that it is a bottomless abyss.

So the amount of steps you take makes no difference. The abyss remains the same. He will lead you along for ninety-nine steps, and you will be very happy – as if you have covered the abyss and now the bottom has come nearer. No, the bottom remains as far away as before. The ninety-nine steps are just to befool your mind, just to give you a "how," a technique. At the hundredth step he says, "Jump!" The abyss remains the same, the span the same.

There is no difference, because the abyss is infinite, God is infinite. How can you meet him gradually? But these ninety-nine steps will befool you. Patanjali is more clever. Heraclitus is innocent, he simply says to you, "This is the thing; here is the abyss. Jump!" He does not persuade you, and he does not seduce you, he simply says, "This is the fact. If you want to jump, jump; if you don't want to jump, go away." He knows that to make steps is useless because finally one has to take the jump. But I think it will be good for you to follow Patanjali because by and by, he seduces you. At least you can take one step and the second becomes easier, then the third. When you have taken ninety-nine steps, it will be difficult to go back because it will be absolutely against your ego – the whole world will laugh. You have become such a great sage, and you are coming back to the world? You were such a *mahayogi* – a great yogi – why are you coming back? Now you are caught, and you cannot go back.

Heraclitus is simple, innocent. His teaching is not that of a kindergarten, but he is a child – that's right – innocent like a child, wise also like a child. Patanjali is cunning, clever. He will suit you because you need somebody who can lead you in a cunning way to a point from where you cannot go back – it becomes simply impossible.

Gurdjieff used to say that there are two types of masters: one innocent and simple; another sly and cunning. He himself said, "I belong to the second category." Patanjali is the source of all sly masters. They lead you to the rose garden and suddenly, the abyss. You are caught in such a grip of your own making that you cannot go back. You meditated, renounced the world, wife and children; for years you were doing postures, meditating, and you created such an aura around you that people worshipped you. Millions of people looked to you as a god – and now comes the abyss. Now, just to save your prestige, you have to jump. Where to go? Now you cannot go anywhere.

Buddha is simple; Patanjali is sly. All science is cunning. This has to be understood, and remember, I am not saying it in any derogatory sense; I am not condemning it. All science is cunning!

It is said that a follower of Lao Tzu – an old farmer – was drawing water from a well. Instead of using bullocks or horses, the old man and his son were working like bullocks and carrying the water out of the well, perspiring, breathing hard. It was difficult.

A follower of Confucius was passing by. He said to the old man, "Haven't you heard? This is very primitive. Why are you wasting your breath? Now bullocks and horses can be used. Haven't you heard that in the towns and cities, nobody is working the way you are working now? It is very primitive. Science has progressed fast."

The old man replied, "Wait, don't talk so loudly. When my son has gone, I will reply." When the son had gone to do some work, he said, "Now, you are a dangerous person. If my son ever hears about this, he will immediately say, 'Okay! Then I don't want to pull this. I can't do this work of a bullock any longer. A bullock is needed.'"

The disciple of Confucius said, "What is wrong in that?"

The old man said, "Everything is wrong in it because it is very cunning. It is deceiving the bullock, it is deceiving the horse. And one thing leads to another. If this boy of mine who is young and not wise discovers that he can be cunning with animals, then he will wonder why he cannot be cunning with man. Once he knows that he can exploit through cunningness, I don't know where he will stop. Please leave, and never come back again on this road. Don't bring such cunning things to this village. We are happy."

Lao Tzu is against science. He says science is cunning. It is deceiving nature, exploiting nature – and through cunning ways, forcing nature. The more scientific a man becomes, the more cunning he becomes; it has to be so. An innocent man cannot be scientific, it is difficult. But man has become cunning and clever, and Patanjali, knowing well that to be scientific is to be cunning, also knows that man can only be brought back to nature through a new device, a new cunningness.

Yoga is the science of the inner being. Because you are not innocent, you have to be brought back to nature through a cunning way. If you are innocent, no means are needed, no methods are needed. A simple understanding, a childlike understanding and you will be transformed. But you are not. That's why you feel that Patanjali seems to be very great. It is because of your head oriented mind and your cunningness.

The second thing to remember is that he appears difficult. You think Heraclitus is simple? Patanjali appears difficult; that too appeals to the ego. The ego always wants to do something which is difficult because against the difficult you feel you are someone. If something is very simple, how can the ego feed off it?

People come to me and say, "Sometimes you teach that just by sitting and doing nothing it can happen. How can it be so simple? How can it be so easy?" Chuang Tzu says, "Easy is right," but these people say, "No! How can it be so easy? It must be difficult – very, very difficult, arduous."

You want to do difficult things because when you are fighting against some difficulty, against the current, you feel you are someone – a conqueror. If something is simple, if something is so easy that even a child can do it, where will your ego stand? You ask for hurdles, you ask for difficulties. And if there are no difficulties you create them so that you can fight, so that you can fly against a strong wind and can feel: "I am someone – a conqueror!" But don't be so smart.

You know the phrase "smart aleck"? You may not know where it comes from – it comes from Alexander. The word *aleck* comes from a short form of Alexander. "Don't be a smart Alexander." Be simple, and don't try to be a conqueror because that is foolish. Don't try to be a somebody.

But Patanjali appealed; Patanjali appealed to the Indian ego very much, so India has created the most subtle egoists in the world. You cannot find anywhere in the world more subtle egoists than you can find in India. It is almost impossible to find a simple yogi. A yogi cannot be simple because he is doing so many asanas, so many mudras, and he is working so hard, how can he be simple? He thinks himself to be at the top – a conqueror. The whole world has to bow down to him; he is the cream – the very salt of life.

Go and watch yogis; you will find that they all have very, very refined egos. Their inner shrine is still empty, the divine has not entered. That shrine is still a throne for their own egos. They may have become very subtle; they may have become so subtle that they may appear to be very humble, but if you watch, you will also find the ego in their humbleness.

They are aware that they are humble, that's the difficulty. A really humble person is not aware that he is humble. A really humble person is simply humble, not aware. And a really humble person never claims that he is humble because all claims are of the ego. Humility cannot be claimed; humbleness is not a claim, it is a state of being. All claims fulfill the ego. Why has this happened? Why has India become a very subtle egoist country? When there is ego, you become blind.

Now when you talk to Indian yogis, they condemn the whole world. They say that the West is materialist; only India is spiritual. The whole world is materialist... As if there is a monopoly. They are so blind that they cannot see that the exact opposite is the case. The more I have been watching the Indian and Western minds, the more I feel the Western mind is less materialist than the Indian. The Indian mind is more materialist, clings to things more, cannot share; it is miserly. The Western mind can share, is less miserly. And because the West has created so much materialist affluence that does not mean it is materialist, and because India is poor that does not mean it is spiritual.

If poverty were spirituality, then impotence would be *brahmacharya*. No, poverty is not spirituality; neither is affluence materialism. Materialism does not belong to things, it belongs to the attitude. Neither does spirituality belong to poverty, it belongs to the inner – a nonattached sharing.

In India you cannot find anybody sharing anything. Nobody can share; everybody hoards, and because they are such hoarders, they are poor. And because a few people hoard too much, many people become poor.

The West has been sharing. That's why the whole society rises from poverty to affluence. In India a few people have become so rich, you cannot find such rich people anywhere else – they are but a few – and the whole society drags itself in poverty. The gap is vast, you cannot find such a gap anywhere. The gap between a wealthy man like Birla and a beggar is vast. Such a gap cannot exist anywhere else, does not exist anywhere else. There are rich and poor people in the West, but the gap is not so vast. Here the gap is simply infinite. You cannot imagine such a gap. How can it be filled? – it cannot be filled because the people are materialist. Otherwise how and why would this gap exist? Can't you share? – impossible! But the ego says that the whole world is materialistic. This has come about because people were attracted to Patanjali and to all the people who were giving difficult methods. There is nothing wrong with Patanjali, but the Indian ego found a beautiful, subtle outlet to be egoistic.

The same is happening to you. Patanjali appeals to you because he is difficult. Heraclitus is "kindergarten" because he is so simple. Simplicity never appeals to the ego. But remember, if simplicity can become an appeal, the path is not long. If difficulty becomes the appeal, the path is going to be very long because from the very beginning, rather than dropping the ego you have started accumulating it.

I am not speaking on Patanjali to make you more egoistic. Look and watch. I am always afraid of talking about Patanjali;

I am never afraid of talking on Heraclitus, Basho, Buddha. I am afraid because of you. Patanjali is beautiful, but you can be attracted for the wrong reasons. This will be a wrong reason, if you think he is difficult – the difficulty of it becomes the attraction.

Edmund Hillary, who conquered Everest – the highest peak, the only peak which was unconquered, was asked, "What is the need to reach the peak? Why do you take so much trouble? And even if you reach it, what will you do then? You will have to come back down again."

Hillary replied, "It is a challenge to the human ego. An unconquered peak has to be conquered!" It had no other utility. What will you do? What has he done? He went there, placed a flag and came back. What nonsense! And many people died in the effort. For almost a hundred years many groups had been trying. Many died, were lost, fell into the abyss – never came back. The more difficult it became to reach, the more it appealed.

Why go to the moon? What will you do there? Isn't the earth enough? But no, the human ego cannot tolerate that the moon remains unconquered. Man must reach there, and because it is so difficult, it has to be conquered. So you can be attracted for the wrong reasons. Now going to the moon is not a poetic effort; it is not like small children who raise their hands and try to catch the moon. And since humanity came into existence every child has longed to reach to the moon. Every child has tried, but the difference must be deeply understood. The effort of a child is beautiful. The moon is so beautiful. It is a poetic effort to touch it, to reach it. There is no ego; it is a simple attraction, a love affair. Every child falls into that love affair. If you can find a child who is not attracted by the moon, what type of child is that?

The moon creates a subtle poetry, a subtle attraction. One would like to touch it and feel it; one would like to go to the moon. But for the scientist that is not the reason. To the scientist, the moon is there as a challenge. How does the moon dare to be continuously there, and to be a challenge? And man is here and he cannot reach it. He has to reach it!

You can be attracted to it for the wrong reasons. The fault is not with the moon; neither is the fault with Patanjali. But you should not be attracted for the wrong reasons. Patanjali is difficult – the most difficult – because he analyzes the whole path, and each fragment seems to be very difficult. But difficulty should not be the appeal: remember that. You can walk through Patanjali's door, but you should not fall in love with the difficulty, but with the insight – the light that Patanjali throws on the path. You should fall in love with the light, not with the difficulty of the path. That will be a wrong reason.

"What you have been saying about Heraclitus, Christ and Zen seems like kindergarten teachings compared to Patanjali." Please don't compare. Comparison is also from the ego. In the real existence, things exist without any comparison. A tree which reaches four hundred feet into the sky and a very, very small grass flower are both the same as far as existence is concerned. But you look and say, "This is a great tree, and what is this? – just ordinary grass." You bring comparison in, and wherever there is comparison, ugliness follows. You have destroyed a beautiful phenomenon.

The tree was great in its "tree-ness" and the grass was great in its "grassiness." The tree may have risen four hundred feet and its flowers may open in the highest sky; the grass is just clinging to the earth and its flowers will be very, very small. Nobody may even be aware when they flower and when they fade. But when this grass flowers, the phenomenon of flowering is the same, the celebration is the same, and there is not a bit of difference. Remember this: that in existence there is no comparison. The mind brings in comparison. It says, "You are more beautiful." Can't you simply say, "You are beautiful"? Why bring in "more"?

Mulla Nasruddin was in love with a woman, and as women

are prone, when Mulla Nasruddin kissed her she asked, "Are you kissing me as the first woman? Am I the first woman you have kissed? Is this the first kiss you have given to a woman?"

Nasruddin said, "Yes, the first and the sweetest."

Comparison is in your blood. You cannot stay with a thing as it is. The woman is also asking for a comparison; otherwise why worry whether this is a first or a second kiss? Each kiss is fresh and virgin. It has no relationship with any kiss from the past or in the future. Each kiss is an existence in itself. It exists alone in its solitariness. It is a peak in itself; it is a unit – not in any way connected with the past or with the future. Why ask whether it is the first? What beauty does the first have? Why not the second or the third?

But the mind wants to compare. Why does the mind want to compare? – because the ego is fed through comparison. It can feel, "I am the first woman; this is the first kiss." You are not interested in the kiss – in the quality of the kiss. This moment the kiss opened a door of your heart; you are not interested in that – that is nothing. You are more interested in whether it is the first or not. The ego is always interested in comparison, and existence knows no comparison. People like Heraclitus and Patanjali live in existence, not in the mind. Don't compare them.

Many people come to me and ask, "Who is greater, Buddha or Christ?" What foolishness to ask! I say to them, "Buddha is greater than Christ, Christ is greater than Buddha." Why do you go on comparing? There is a subtle thing working: if you are a follower of Christ, you would like Christ to be the greatest because you can only be great if Christ is the greatest. It is a fulfillment of your own ego. How can your master not be the greatest? He has to be because you are such a great disciple. If Christ is not the greatest, where will Christians be? If Buddha is not the greatest, what will happen to the ego of the Buddhists?

Every race, religion, country, thinks itself to be the greatest –

not because any country is great, not because any race is great. In this existence everything is the greatest. Existence creates only the greatest; every being is unique. But that doesn't appeal to the mind because then greatness is so common. Everybody is great? So what is the use of it? Somebody has to be lower. A hierarchy has to be created.

Just the other night I was reading a book by George Mikes and he said that where he was born in Budapest, Hungary, an English woman fell in love with him. He wasn't very much in love with her, but he didn't want to be rude either, so when she asked, "Can we get married?"

He replied, "It will be difficult because my mother will not allow it and she will not be happy if I marry a foreigner."

The English lady was very offended and said, "What? I, a foreigner? I am not a foreigner! I am English! You are a foreigner and your mother too!"

Mikes said, "In Budapest, Hungary, I am a foreigner?"

The woman replied, "Yes! Truth does not depend on geography."

Everyone thinks that way. The mind tries to fulfill its desires, to be the most supreme. One has to be watchful with religion, race, country, everything – very watchful. Only then you can get beyond this subtle phenomenon of the ego.

You say: "Heraclitus, Christ, and Zen make the final step seem close; Patanjali makes even the first step seem almost impossible." That's because it is both. The Upanishad says: "He is closer than the closest and he is farther than the farthest." He is both near and far. He has to be, otherwise who will be far? He has to be near also, otherwise who will be near you? He touches your skin and he is spread beyond the boundaries. He is both!

Heraclitus emphasizes the nearness because he is a simple man. He says that he is so near, nothing is needed to be done to bring him nearer. He is almost there; he is just watching at the gate, knocking at your door, waiting near your heart. Nothing is to be done. Simply be silent and have a look, just sit silently and look. You have never lost him. The truth is near.

In fact, to say that truth is near is wrong because you are also truth. Even nearness seems to be very, very far; even nearness shows that there is a distinction, a distance, a gap. Even that gap is not there – you are it! The Upanishad says, "Thou art that: *tattvamasi Svetketu.*" You are already that; there is not even that much distance to say that he is close. And Heraclitus and Zen both want you to take the jump immediately – not wait.

Patanjali says that he is very far. He is also right, he is also very far. He will appeal to you more, because if he is so close and you have not attained, you will feel very, very depressed. If he is so close, just standing by the side of you; if he is the only neighbor surrounding you from every side and you have not achieved, your ego will feel very, very frustrated. Such a great man like you, and he is so near and you are missing? That seems very frustrating. But if he is very far, everything is okay because time is needed, effort is needed – nothing is wrong with you; he is so far away.

Distance is such a vast thing. You will take some time, and then one day you will get up, move, and you will achieve. If he is near, you will feel guilty and wonder why you are not achieving anything with him? One feels uncomfortable reading Heraclitus, Basho, Buddha. That never happens with Patanjali. One feels at ease.

Look at the paradox of the mind: with the easiest of people one feels uncomfortable. The discomfort comes from you. To move with Heraclitus or Jesus is very uncomfortable because they go on insisting that the kingdom of God is within you – and you know that nothing exists within you except hell. They insist that the kingdom of God is within you; it becomes uncomfortable.

If the kingdom of God is within you, then something must be wrong with you. Why can't you see it? If it is so present, why can't it happen right this moment? That is the message of Zen – that it is immediate. There is no need to wait, no need to waste time. It can happen right now, this very moment! There is no excuse. This makes you uncomfortable; you feel uncomfortable, you cannot find any excuse. With Patanjali, you can find millions of excuses. He is very far, and millions of lives' effort is needed. Yes, it can be attained, but always in the future. You are at ease. There is no urgency about it, and you can be as you are right now. Tomorrow morning you will start moving on the path – and tomorrow never comes.

Patanjali gives you space, gives you future. He says, "Do this and that, and by and by you will attain – some day, nobody knows, in some future life…" You are at ease, there is no urgency. You can be as you are; there is no hurry.

These Zen people, they drive you crazy! And I drive you even crazier because I talk from both sides. This is just a way. This is a koan. This is just a way to drive you crazy. I use Heraclitus, I use Patanjali, but these are tricks to drive you crazy. You simply cannot be allowed to relax. Whenever there is a future, you are okay. The mind can desire God, and nothing is wrong with you. The very phenomenon is such that it will take time. This becomes an excuse.

With Patanjali you can postpone, with Zen you cannot. If you do postpone, it is you who are postponing, not God. With Patanjali you can postpone because the very nature of God is such that it can be attained only in gradual ways. It is very, very difficult. That is why you feel comfortable with difficulty. This is the paradox: with people who say that it is easy, you feel uncomfortable; with people who say it is difficult, you feel comfortable. It should be just the opposite.

The truth is both, so it depends on you. If you want to postpone, Patanjali is perfect. If you want it here and now, you will have to listen to Zen and you will have to decide. Are you feeling the urgency? Haven't you suffered enough? Or do you want to suffer more? Then Patanjali is perfect – follow Patanjali. And somewhere in the distant future you will attain bliss. But if you have suffered enough... And this is what maturity is: understanding that you have suffered enough.

You call Heraclitus and Zen for children? Kindergarten? This is the only maturity, to have been realized: "I have suffered enough." If you feel this, an urgency is created, a fire is created. Something has to be done right now! You cannot postpone it; there is no meaning in postponing. You have postponed it enough already. But if you want it in the future, if you would like to suffer a little more, if you have become addicted to the hell – to remain the same just one more day – or if you would like some modifications, follow Patanjali.

That is what Patanjali says: "Do this and do that, slowly. Do one thing, and then another thing." And millions of things have to be done and they cannot be done immediately, so you go on modifying yourself. Today you take a vow that you will be non-violent, and tomorrow you will take another vow. The day after tomorrow you will become celibate... In this way it goes on and on. There are millions of things to leave behind: lying, violence, aggression, all have to be dropped; by and by anger, hate, jealousy, possessiveness – millions of things. Meanwhile, you remain the same.

How can you drop anger if you have not dropped hate? How can you drop anger if you have not dropped jealousy? How can you drop anger if you have not dropped aggressiveness? They are interrelated.

So you say that now you will no longer be angry. What are you talking about? Nonsense! You will remain hateful, you will remain aggressive. You would still like to dominate, you would still love to be at the top – and you are dropping anger? How you can drop it? They are interrelated.

This is what Zen says: "If you want to drop it, understand the phenomenon that everything is related." Either you drop it now or you never drop it. Don't befool yourself. You can simply whitewash over it – a little here, a patch there, and the old house remains with all its oldness. While you go on working, painting the walls and filling the holes, this and that, you think you are creating a new life and meanwhile you continue in the same way. The more you continue, the more it becomes deep-rooted.

Don't deceive yourself. If you can understand, it is immediate. That is the message of Zen. If you cannot understand, something has to be done, and Patanjali will be good – so follow Patanjali. One day or other you will have to come to an understanding and you will see that this whole thing has been a trick – a trick of your mind to avoid the reality, to avoid and escape – and on that day, suddenly you will drop it.

Patanjali is gradual, Zen is sudden. If you cannot be sudden, it is better to be gradual. Rather than being nothing, neither this nor that, it is better to be gradual. Patanjali will also bring you to the same situation, but he will give you a little space. It is more comfortable – difficult, but more comfortable. No immediate transformation is demanded. The mind can fit in with a gradual progress.

You say: "Heraclitus, Christ, and Zen make the final step seem close; Patanjali makes even the first step seem almost impossible. It seems like we Westerners have hardly begun to realize the amount of work that has to be done." It is up to you. If you want to do the work, you can do it. If you want to realize without doing the work, that too is possible. That too is possible! It is up to you to choose. If you want to do hard work, I will give you hard work. I can create even more steps. Patanjali can be stretched even longer. I can put the goal even farther away; I can give you impossible things to do. It is your choice. Or if you really want to realize, this can be done this very moment. It is up to you. Patanjali is a way of looking, Heraclitus is also a way of looking.

Once it happened...

I was walking along a street and saw a small child eating a very big watermelon. The melon was too big for him. I looked and watched and saw that he was finding it a little difficult to finish it. So I said to him, "It seems to be really too big, don't you think?"

The boy looked at me and said, "No! There is not enough me."

He is also right. Everything can be looked at from two standpoints. God is near and far. Now it is for you to decide where you would like to take the jump from – near or far. If you want to take the jump from far, then all the techniques come in because they will take you far – from there you will take the jump. It is just like you are standing on this shore of the ocean; the ocean is here, and also there at the other shore – which is completely invisible, very, very far away. You can take the jump from this shore because it is the same ocean, but if you decide to take the jump from the other shore, Patanjali gives you a boat.

The whole of Yoga is a boat to go to the other shore to take the jump. It is up to you. You can enjoy the journey; there is nothing wrong in it. I am not saying it is wrong; it is up to you. You can take the boat and go to the other shore and take the jump from there. But the same ocean exists here. Why not take the jump from this shore? The jump will be the same, the ocean will be the same, and you will be the same. What difference does it make if you go to the other shore? There may be people on the other shore who may be trying to come here. And there are Patanjalis there who have also made boats. They are coming here to take the jump from the far away.

It happened...

A man was trying to cross a road. It was the rush hour, and it was difficult to cross. Cars were going so fast, and he was a very, very mild mannered man. He tried many times and came back. Then he saw an old acquaintance, Mulla Nasruddin, on the

other side. He cried, "Nasruddin, how did you cross the road?"
Nasruddin replied, "I never crossed it. I was born on this side."

There are people who are always thinking of the distant shore.
The distant always looks beautiful; the distant has a magnetism of
its own because it is covered in mist. But the ocean is the same. It
is up to you to choose. Nothing is wrong in going on that ocean,
but go for the right reasons. You may be simply avoiding the
jump from this shore. And even if the boat leads you to the other
shore, the moment you reach it you will start thinking of this shore
because this will be the faraway point. Many times, in many lives,
you have done this. You have changed the shore, but you have
not taken the jump.

I have seen you crossing the ocean from this side to that and
from that side to this. This is the problem: that shore is far away
because you are here. When you are there, this shore will be far
away. You are in such a sleep you have completely forgotten that
you have also been to that shore again and again. By the time you
reach the other shore, you have forgotten the shore that you have
left behind. By the time you reach it, oblivion takes over.

You look to the distant shore and again somebody says, "Here
is a boat, sir. You can go to the other shore and take the jump
from there because God is very, very far away." Again you start
the preparation to leave this shore. Patanjali gives you a boat to go
to the other shore, but when you have reached there, Zen will
always give you the jump. The final jump is of Zen. Meanwhile
you can do many things; that is not the point. Whenever you take
the jump it will be a sudden jump, it cannot be gradual.

All gradualness is in going from this shore to that – but
nothing is wrong in it. If you enjoy the journey, it is beautiful
because he is here, he is in the middle, and also at that shore. No
need to reach to the other shore either. You can take the jump in
the middle, just from the boat. The boat becomes the shore.
Where ever you jump from is the shore. Every moment, where

ever you can take the jump from becomes the shore. If you don't take the jump, it is no longer the shore. It depends on you; remember this well.

That's why I am talking about all the contradictory standpoints, so that you can understand from every side. You can see the reality from every side and you can decide. If you decide to wait a little, beautiful. If you decide to take the jump right now, beautiful. To me everything is beautiful and great, and I have no choice. I simply give you all the choices. If you say, "I would like to wait a little," I say, "Good! I bless you. Wait a little." If you say, "I am ready and I want to jump," I say, "Jump, with my blessings."

For me there is no choice – neither Heraclitus, nor Patanjali. I am simply opening all the doors for you with the hope that you may enter a door. But remember the tricks of the mind. When I talk about Heraclitus you think it is too vague, too mysterious, too simple. When I talk about Patanjali you think it is too difficult, almost impossible. I open the door and you interpret something and make a judgment and stop yourself. The door is not open for you to judge, the door is open for you to enter.

The second question:

Osho,
You talked of moving from faith to trust. How can we
use the mind that swings from doubt to belief to go
beyond these two polarities?

Doubt and belief are not different – both are aspects of the same coin. This has to be understood first because people think that when they believe, they have gone beyond doubt. Belief is the same as doubt because both are concerns of the mind. Your mind argues, says no, finds no proof to say yes – and you doubt. Your mind then finds arguments to say yes, proof to say yes – and you believe. In both cases you believe in reason; in both cases you believe in arguments. The difference is on the surface. Deep down you believe in the reasoning. Trust is the dropping out of reasoning. It is mad, irrational, absurd.

I say that trust is not faith. Trust is a personal encounter. Faith is again given and borrowed. It is a conditioning. Faith is a conditioning which your parents, your culture, and society give you. You don't bother about it; you don't make it a personal concern. It is a given thing. A thing which is given and which has not been a personal growth is just a facade, a false face, a Sunday face.

For six days of the week you are different; then on Sunday you enter the church and you put on a mask. See how people behave in church: so gently, so humanly – the same people! Even a murderer goes to church and prays. Look at his face – it looks so beautiful, so innocent, and this man has killed! In church you have a proper face to use and you know how to use it. It's a conditioning. It is given to you in your very childhood.

Faith is given; trust is a growth.

You encounter reality, you face it, you live it, and by and by you come to an understanding that doubt leads to hell, to misery. The more you doubt, the more miserable you become. If you doubt completely, you will be in perfect misery. If you are not in perfect misery, that is because you cannot doubt completely. You still trust. Even an atheist trusts. Even a man who doubts whether the world exists or not also trusts; otherwise he cannot live, and life will become impossible.

If doubt becomes total, you cannot live for a single moment more. How can you breathe in, if you doubt? If you really doubt, who knows if the breath isn't poisonous? Who knows, maybe millions of germs are being carried in? And who knows, maybe cancer is being carried in with the breath?

If you really doubt, you cannot even breathe. You cannot live for a single moment more; you will die immediately. Doubt is suicide, but you never doubt perfectly, so you linger on. You linger on, somehow you drag on. Your life is not total. Just think: if total doubt is suicide, then total trust will be the absolute life possible.

That's what happens to a man of trust: he trusts, and the more he trusts, the more he becomes capable of trusting. The more he becomes capable of trust, the more life opens. He feels more, he lives more, he lives intensely. Life becomes an authentic bliss. Now he can trust more. Not that he is never deceived because if you trust, that doesn't mean that nobody is going to deceive you. In fact, more people will deceive you because you become vulnerable. If you trust, more people will deceive you, but nobody can make you miserable; that is the point to understand. They can deceive you, steal things from you, borrow money and never return it, but nobody can make you miserable. That becomes impossible. Even if they kill you, they cannot make you miserable.

You trust, and it makes you vulnerable, but also absolutely victorious because nobody can defeat you. They can deceive you, they can steal from you and you may become a beggar, but still you will be an emperor.

Trust makes emperors out of beggars and doubt makes beggars out of emperors. Look at an emperor who cannot trust; he is always afraid. He cannot trust his own wife, or children because a king possesses so much that his son will kill him for it, his wife will poison him for it. He cannot trust anybody. He lives in such distrust that he is already in hell. Even when he sleeps he cannot relax. Who knows what is going to happen?

Trust makes you more and more open. Of course, when you are open many things will become possible. When you are open, friends will reach your heart; of course, enemies can also reach your heart... The door is open. So there are two possibilities. If you want to be secure, you close the door completely. Bolt it, lock it and hide inside. Now no enemy can enter, but neither can a friend. Even if God comes, he cannot enter. Now nobody can deceive you, but what is the point? You are in a grave. You are already dead. Nobody can kill you, but you are already dead; you cannot come out. Of course, you live in security, but what type of life is this? You don't live at all.

Then you open the door. Doubt is closing the door; trust is opening it. When you open the door, all the alternatives become possible. Friends may enter, foes may enter. The wind will come, and bring the perfume of flowers. It will also bring the germs of diseases. Now everything is possible – the good and the bad. Love will come; hate will also come. Now God can come and also the Devil. This is the fear – that something may go wrong; so you close the door. But then everything goes wrong. Open the door – there is a possibility that something can go wrong, but if your trust is total, not for you. You will find a friend even in the enemy, you will find God even in the Devil. Trust is such a trans-formation, your whole outlook changes and you cannot find anything bad.

That is the meaning of Jesus' saying, "Love your enemies." How can you love your enemies? It has been a problem to be solved – an enigma for Christian theologians. How can you love your enemy? But a man of trust can because a man of trust knows no enemies. A man of trust knows only the friend. It makes no difference in what form he comes. If he comes to steal, he is a friend; if he comes to take, he is a friend; if he comes to give, he is a friend – in whatever form he comes.

Once it happened that al-Hillaj Mansoor, a great mystic and Sufi, was murdered, killed, crucified. His last words, as he looked at the sky, were: "But you cannot deceive me." Many people were there; al-Hillaj was smiling and he said in the direction of the sky, "Look, you cannot deceive me."

So somebody asked, "What do you mean? Who are you talking to?"

He replied, "I am talking to my God; in whatever form you come you cannot deceive me. I know you well. Now you have come as death. You cannot deceive me."

A man of trust cannot be deceived. In whatever form, whoever comes, it is always the divine coming to him, because trust makes everything holy. Trust is an alchemy. It transforms not only you, it transforms the whole world for you. Wherever you look you find him; in the friend, in the foe; in the night, in the day. Yes, Heraclitus is right: "God is summer and winter, day and night; God is satiety and hunger." This is trust. Patanjali makes trust the base – the base of all growth.

You say: "You talked of moving from faith to trust..." Faith is that which is given; trust is that which is found. Faith is given by your parents; trust has to be found by you. Faith is given by the society; to find trust you have to search, seek, inquire. Trust is personal, intimate; faith is like a commodity – you can purchase it in the market.

You can purchase it in the market – when I say it, I say it with a very considered mind. You can become a Mohammedan, you can become a Hindu. Go into an Arya temple and you can be converted to a Hindu. There's no problem. Faith can be purchased in the market. From being a Mohammedan you can become a Hindu, from being a Hindu you can become a Jaina. It is so simple that any foolish priest can do it. But trust is not a commodity. You can't go and find it in the market; you cannot purchase it. You have to pass through many experiences. By and by it arises, by and by it changes you. A new quality, a new flame comes to your being.

So when you see that doubt is misery, trust comes. When you see that faith is dead, trust comes. Being a Christian, Hindu, Mohammedan, have you ever observed the fact that you are completely dead? What type of Christian are you? If you are really a Christian you will be a Christ – nothing less than that. Trust will make you a Christ; faith will make you a Christian – a very poor substitute. You go to church, you read the Bible – so what type of Christian are you? – your faith is not a knowing, it is an ignorance.

It happened...

A great economist came to talk at a Rotary Club. He talked in the jargon of economists. The local priest was also present to listen to him. After the talk, he approached the economist and said, "You gave a beautiful talk, but to be frank, I couldn't follow a single word."

The economist replied, "In that case, I would say to you what you say to your listeners: 'Have faith!'"

When you cannot understand, when you are ignorant, the whole society says, "Have faith." I say to you that it is better to doubt than to have a false faith. It is better to doubt because doubt will create misery. Faith is a consolation; doubt will create misery. If there is misery, you will have to seek trust. This is the problem, the dilemma that has happened in the world – because of faith, you have forgotten how to seek trust; because of faith, you have become trustless; because of faith, you are carrying corpses. You are Christians, Hindus, Mohammedans, and you miss the whole point. And because of faith, you think you are religious. Then the inquiry stops.

Honest doubt is better than dishonest faith.

All faith is false if you have not grown into it, if it is not your feeling, your being, your experience. All faith is false. Be honest. Doubt! Suffer! Only suffering will bring you to understanding. If you truly suffer, one day or other you will understand that it is doubt that is making you suffer. Transformation then becomes possible.

You ask me, "How can we use the mind that swings from doubt to belief to go beyond these two polarities?" You cannot use it because you have never been an honest doubter. Your faith is false, with doubt hidden deep down. Just on the surface there is a whitewash of faith. Deep down you are doubtful, but you are afraid to know that you are doubtful, so you go on clinging to faith, you go on making gestures of faith. You can make gestures, but through gestures you cannot attain reality. You can bow down at a shrine; you are making the gesture of a man who trusts, but you will not grow because deep down there is no trust, only doubt. Faith is just superimposed.

It is just like kissing a person you don't love. From the outside everything is the same; you are making the gesture of kissing. No scientist can find any difference. If you kiss a person, the photograph of the kiss, the physiological phenomenon, the transfer of millions of germs from one lip to another, everything is exactly the same whether you love the person or not. If a scientist watches and observes, what will the difference be? – no difference, not a single iota of difference. He will say both are kisses and are exactly the same.

But you know when you love a person, something of the invisible passes which cannot be detected by any instrument. When you don't love a person, you can kiss but nothing passes between you – no energy communication, no communion happens. It is exactly the same with faith and trust. Trust is a kiss with love, with a deeply loving heart; faith is a kiss without any love.

So from where to begin? – the first thing is to inquire into doubt. Throw away the false faith, and become an honest, sincere doubter. Your sincerity will help because if you are honest, how can you miss the point that doubt creates suffering? If you are sincere, you are bound to know. Sooner or later you will come to realize that doubt has been creating more misery – the more you go into doubt, the more misery you feel. One grows only through misery.

When you come to a point where misery becomes impossible to tolerate, you drop it. Not that you really drop it; the very intolerability becomes the dropping. Once there is no more doubt and you have suffered through it, you start moving toward trust.

Trust, *shraddha*, is transformation. And Patanjali says that *shraddha*, trust, is the very base of all *samadhi*, of all ultimate experience of the divine.

Enough for today.

3

With Both Effort or Surrender, Totality Is Needed

Success is nearest to those whose efforts are intense
and sincere.

The chances of success vary according to the degree
of effort.

Success is also attained by those who
surrender to God.

God is the supreme ruler.

He is an individual unit of divine consciousness.
He is untouched by the afflictions of life,
action and its result.

In God the seed is developed to its highest extent.

There are three types of seekers. The first type comes onto the path because of curiosity. Patanjali calls it *kutuhal*. This type is not really interested; he has drifted into it as if by accident. He may have read something, he may have heard somebody talk about God, truth, the ultimate liberation, and became interested. The interest is intellectual, just like a child who becomes interested in each and every thing and after a time, averts his attention as more and more curiosities are always opening their doors.

Such a man will never attain. You cannot attain the truth out of curiosity because truth needs a persistent effort, a continuity, a perseverance which a man of curiosity cannot have. A man of curiosity can do a certain thing for a certain period of time according to his mood, but then there is a gap and all that he has done disappears, is undone. He will start again from the very beginning, and the same will happen.

He cannot reap the result. He can sow the seeds, but cannot wait because millions of new interests are always calling him. He goes to the south, he moves to the east; he goes to the west, then to the north. He is like wood drifting in the sea; he is not going anywhere. His energy is not moving toward a certain goal. Whatever circumstance pushes him… He is accidental, and the accidental man cannot attain the divine. He may be very active, but it is all futile because in the day he will do it and in the night he will undo it. Perseverance is needed; a continuous hammering is needed.

Jalaluddin Rumi had a small school – a school of wisdom. He used to take his disciples to the fields, to the farms around about. He used to take all his new disciples to one particular farm, in order to show them what happened there. Whenever a new disciple came, he would take him to that farm. There was something worthwhile there; the farmer was an example of a certain state of mind. He would dig a well, ten, fifteen feet, and then he would change his mind saying, "This place doesn't look good." So he would start another hole, and then another.

He had been doing it for many years. And at that time there were eight incomplete holes. The whole farm was destroyed, and he was working on the ninth. Jalaluddin would say to his new disciples, "Look! Don't be like this farmer. If he had put all his effort into one hole, by this time it would have been at least one hundred feet deep. He has made so much effort, and been very active, but he cannot wait. He digs for ten, twelve, fifteen feet, gets bored, and starts another hole. This way the whole farm will be covered with holes, and there will never be a well."

This is the man of curiosity, the accidental man who, when he does things, starts with so much zeal – in fact, too much. And too much zeal cannot become a continuity. He starts with such vigor and zest that you know that soon he will have to stop.

The second type of man who comes to the inner search is the man of *jigyasa* – inquiry. He has not come out of curiosity, he has come with an intense inquiry. He means it, but it is also not enough because his meaning is basically intellectual. He may become a philosopher, but he cannot become a religious man. He inquires deeply, but his inquiry is intellectual. It remains head-oriented; it is a problem to be solved.

Life and death are not involved; it is not a question of life and death. It is a riddle, a puzzle. He enjoys solving it, just as you enjoy solving a crossword puzzle because it gives you a challenge. It has to be solved, and you will feel very good if you solve it. But this is intellectual, and deep down, the ego is involved. This man becomes a philosopher. He tries hard. He thinks, he contemplates, but he never meditates – he reflects logically, rationally and finds many clues. He creates a system, but the whole thing is his own projection.

Truth needs your totality. Even ninety-nine percent won't do; exactly one hundred percent of you is needed, and the head is only one percent. You can live without the head. Animals are living without the head, trees are living without the head. In existence, a head is not such an essential thing. You can easily live... In fact, you can live more easily without the head than you can with it. It creates millions of complexities. A head is just not an absolute necessity, and nature knows that. It is a superfluous luxury. If you don't have enough food, the body knows where the food should go – it stops giving it to the head.

That's why the intellect cannot develop in poor countries – intellect is a luxury. When everything is finished, and the body is getting completely everything, only then does the energy move toward the head. It happens every day even in your own life, but you are not aware of it. If you eat too much food, you immediately feel sleepy. What is happening? – the body needs energy for digestion. The head can be forgotten; the energy moves toward the stomach. The head feels dizzy, sleepy. The energy is not moving, blood is not moving toward the head. The body has its own economy.

There are basic things, there are non-basic things. Basic things have to be fulfilled first because the non-basic can wait – your philosophy can wait, there is not much of a need for it. But your stomach cannot wait, it has to be fulfilled first; that hunger is more basic. Many religions have tried fasting because of this basic realization – if you fast the head cannot think. There is not so much energy, so it cannot be given to the head. But this is a deception. When the energy returns there again, the head will start thinking once more. This type of meditation is a lie.

If you fast for a longer time, continuously for a few days, the head cannot think. It is not that you have attained no-mind, now there is simply no superfluous energy in you. The body's needs are first – bodily needs are basic, essential; the head's needs are secondary, superfluous. It is just the same as when you make an economy in your home; if your child is dying you will sell the TV set. There is nothing much involved in it. You can sell the furniture when the child is dying; you can even sell the house, when you are hungry. First things first – that is the meaning of economy – second things second. And the head is the last; it is only one percent of you, and that too is superfluous. You can exist without it.

Can you exist without the stomach? Can you exist without the heart? But you *can* exist without the head. When you pay too much attention to the head, you are completely upside down. You are doing *shirshasan*: standing on the head. You have completely forgotten that a head is not essential. When you give only your head to an inquiry, it is *jigyasa*. It is a luxury. You can become a philosopher and sit in an armchair, rest and think. Philosophers are like luxurious furniture. If you can afford it, good, but it is not a life-and-death situation. So Patanjali says, "The man of *kutuhal*, the man of curiosity, cannot achieve; the man of *jigyasa*, inquiry, will become a philosopher."

There is the third man whom Patanjali calls, "The man of *mumuksha*." This word *mumuksha* is difficult to translate, so I will explain it: *Mumuksha* means the desire to be desireless. The desire to be completely liberated, and to get out of the wheel of existence; not to be born again, not to die again. The feeling that it is enough – born millions of times, dying again and again, moving in the same vicious circle. *Mumuksha* means to become the ultimate dropout, from the very wheel of existence – bored, suffering, one wants to get out of it. The inquiry now becomes a life-and-death situation. Your whole being is at stake. Patanjali says that only a man of *mumuksha* – in whom the desire for *moksha*, liberation, has arisen – can become a religious man because he is a very, very logical thinker.

There are also three types of men who belong to the category of *mumuksha*. The first type of man who belongs to *mumuksha* puts one-third of his being into the effort. In putting one-third of your being into the effort you will attain something. What you attain will be a negative achievement; you will not be tense – this has to be understood very deeply – but you will not be calm either. You will not be tense – tensions drop – but you will not be tranquil, calm, cool. The attainment will be negative. You will not be ill, but you will not be healthy either. Illness will disappear. You will not feel irritated or frustrated, but you will not feel fulfilled either. The negative will drop, the thorns will drop, but the flower will not appear.

This is the first degree of *mumuksha*. You can find many people who are stuck there. You will feel a certain quality in them; they don't react or get irritated, and you cannot make them angry or make them anxious. They have attained something, but you still feel that something is lacking. They are not at ease – even non-angry; they don't have compassion. They may not be angry at you, but they cannot forgive. The difference is subtle. They are not angry, that is right, but even in their being non-angry there is no forgiveness. They are stuck.

They don't bother about you or your insult; in a way, they are cut off from all relating. They can't share, and in trying not to be angry, they have moved away from all relationships. They have become like islands – closed. And when you are an island, closed, you are uprooted. You cannot flower, cannot be happy, and cannot have a well-being. It is a negative achievement. Something has been thrown out, but nothing has been attained. Of course, the path is clear. Even to throw something out is very good because now the possibility exists that you can attain something.

Patanjali calls them *mridu*, soft. The first degree of attainment, negative. You will find many sannyasins in India, many monks in Catholic monasteries, who are stuck at the first degree. They are good people, but you will find them dull. It is very good not to be angry, but it is not enough. Something is missing; nothing positive has happened. They are empty vessels. They have emptied themselves, but somehow have not been refilled. The higher has not descended, but the lower has been thrown out.

There is a second degree of *mumuksha* – the second degree of the right seeker – who puts two-thirds of himself into the effort. Not yet total, he is just in the middle. Because of the middle, Patanjali calls him *madhya* – the middle man. He attains something. The first-degree man is in him, but something more is added. He is at peace – silent, cool, collected. Whatever happens in the world does not affect him. He remains unaffected, detached. He becomes like a peak: very peaceful.

If you come close to him you feel his peace surrounding you; just as you go into a garden: the cool air, the fragrance of the flowers, the singing of the birds, all surround you. They touch you and you feel them. With the first-degree man, the *mridu*, you will not feel anything, only an emptiness – a desertlike being. The first type of man will suck you in. If you go near him you will feel that you have been emptied – that somebody has been sucking you in, because he is a desert. With him you will feel yourself being dried out, and you will be afraid.

You will feel this with many sannyasins. If you go near them you feel they are sucking you, not knowingly. They have attained the first degree. They have become empty, and that very emptiness becomes like a hole and you are automatically sucked in by it.

It is said that in Tibet this first-degree man, where ever he is, should not be allowed to move about in the town. When lamas in Tibet attain the first degree they are prohibited from leaving the monasteries – because if the man comes in contact with any-body, he sucks. That sucking is beyond his control; he cannot do anything about it. He is like a desert. Anything that comes near him becomes sucked, exploited.

First-degree lamas are not allowed to touch a tree because it has been observed that the tree dies. Even in the Himalayas, a Hindu sannyasin is not allowed to touch trees – they will die. He is a sucking phenomenon. This first-degree lama is not allowed to attend anybody's marriage because he will become a destructive force. He is not allowed to bless anybody because he cannot bless. Even when he is blessing, he is sucking. You may not have known it, but monasteries were created for these first-degree lamas, san-nyasins, sadhus, so that they can live in an enclosed world of their own. They are not allowed to move out. They are not allowed to bless anybody, unless they attain the second degree.

The second-degree seeker, who has put in two-thirds of his being, becomes peaceful, calm. If you go near him, he flows into you, he shares. Now he is no longer a desert; now he is a green forest. Many things are arising in him – he is silent, calm, tran-quil. You will feel it. But this is also not the goal, and many become stuck there. Just to be silent is not enough. What type of achievement is this? Just to be silent? It is like death – no move-ment, no activity. You are at peace of course, at home of course, but no celebration, no bliss.

A third-degree seeker, who puts his totality into it, attains bliss. Bliss is a positive phenomenon; peace is just on the way. When bliss comes nearer, the second-degree seeker become peaceful. It is a distant influence of the bliss that is reaching close to you. It is just like when you come close to a river: from quite some distance away you start feeling that the air is cooling, that the quality of the greenery is changing. The trees are greener with more foliage; the air is cool. You haven't seen the river yet, but it is somewhere near; the source of water is somewhere near. When the source of life is somewhere near, you become peaceful, but you have not attained yet – it is just on the way. Patanjali calls this man the *madhya*, the middle man.

He is also not the goal. Unless you can dance with ecstasy… This man cannot dance, and he cannot sing because singing will look like you are disturbing the peace, dancing will look foolish – what are you doing? This man can only sit like a dead statue – silent, of course, but not flowering; green, but the flowers haven't happened yet. The final part has not descended.

Then there is the third-degree man, who can dance, who will look mad because he has got so much. He cannot contain it, and because he cannot contain it, he will sing and dance. He will move and share, and wherever he can he will throw the seeds that are showering on him endlessly. This is the third-degree man.

Patanjali says:

> Success is nearest to those whose efforts are intense and sincere.

> The chances of success vary according to the degree of effort.

Success is nearest to those whose efforts are intense and sincere. Your totality is needed. And remember, sincerity is a quality that happens whenever you are in something totally. But people are almost always wrong about their idea of sincerity, they think to be serious is sincere. To be serious is not to be sincere; sincerity is a quality which happens whenever you are in something totally. A child playing with his toys is sincere – totally in it, absorbed, nothing left behind, no holding back; he is not there really, only the play goes on.

If you don't hold anything back, where are you? You have become completely one with the activity. The actor is no longer there, the doer is no longer there. When the doer is not, there is sincerity. How can you be serious? Seriousness belongs to the doer. So in mosques, temples, churches, you will find two types of people – the sincere and the serious. The serious will be there with long faces, as if they are doing a very great thing – something sacred, of the other world. This too is the ego, as if you are doing something great, as if you are obliging the whole world because you are praying.

Look at the religious people – so-called, of course; they walk in such a way as if they are obliging the whole world, that they are the salt of the earth. If they disappear, the whole of existence will disappear. They are supporting it. It is because of them that life exists – because of their prayers. You will find them all serious.

Seriousness belongs to the ego, the doer. Look at a father working in a shop or in an office somewhere. If he doesn't love his wife and children, he will be serious because it is a duty. He is doing it, and obliging everybody around him. He always says, "I am doing it for my wife and children." With his seriousness, this man will become a dead weight hanging around the necks of his children. And they will never be able to forgive him because he never loved them.

If you love, you never say such words. If you love your children you go dancing to your office. You love them; it is not that you are obliging them. You are not fulfilling a duty; it is your love. You are happy that you are allowed to do something for your children. You are happy and blissful that you can do something for your wife because love feels so helpless; love wants to do so many things and cannot. Love always feels, "Whatever I am doing is less than what should be done." And duty? – duty always feels, "I am doing more than is needed." Duty becomes serious; love is sincere. Love is to be totally with a person, to be so totally with a person that the duality disappears. If even for moments there is no duality, one exists in two, a bridge is there. Love is sincere, never serious. And wherever you put your total being in anything, it becomes a love. If you are a gardener and you love, and bring your total being into it – sincerity happens.

You cannot cultivate sincerity. You can cultivate seriousness, but sincerity – no. Sincerity is a shadow of being total in something.

Patanjali says: *Success is nearest to those whose efforts are intense and sincere.* Of course, there is no need to say ...*intense and sincere.* Sincerity is always intense. Why does Patanjali say ...*intense and sincere?* – for a certain reason: sincerity is always intense, but intensity is not necessarily always sincere. You can be intense in something but not sincere, may not be sincere. Hence he adds the qualification ...*intense and sincere,* because you can be intense even in your seriousness. You can be intense even with your partial being, you can be intense in a certain mood; you can be intense in your anger, you can be intense in your lust. You can be intense in millions of things and may not be sincere because sincerity belongs to when you are totally in it.

You can be intense in sex, but you may not be sincere because sex is not necessarily love. You may be very, very intense in your sexuality – but once your sexuality is fulfilled, it is finished, the intensity gone. Love may not look so intense, but it is sincere – and because it is sincere, the intensity continues. In fact, if you are really in love it becomes a timelessness. It is always intense. And make a clear distinction: if you are intense without sincerity, you cannot be intense forever. You can be intense only momentarily; when the desire arises you are intense. It is not really your intensity, it is enforced by the desire.

Sex arises and you feel a starvation, a hunger. The whole body, the whole bioenergy needs a release; you become intense. But this intensity is not yours; it is not coming from your being. It is just enforced by the biological crust around you; it is a bodily enforcement on your being. It is not coming from the center, it is being forced from the periphery. You will be intense, sex is fulfilled, and the intensity gone... Then you don't care about the woman.

Many women have told me that they feel cheated, deceived, used because in the beginning when their husbands make love to them, they feel so loving, so intense, so happy. The moment sex is finished, the men turn over and go to sleep. They don't care at all what happens to the woman. After you have made love you don't even say good-bye, you don't thank the woman; she feels used.

Your intensity is biological, bodily; it is not coming from you. In the intensity of sex there is a foreplay, but no afterplay. The word doesn't really exist. I have seen thousands of books written on sex; the word *afterplay* doesn't exist. What type of love is this? Bodily needs fulfilled – finished! The woman feels she has been used; now you can discard her. Just as you use something and throw it away, like a plastic container – you use it and throw it away. Finished! When the desire arises again, you look at the woman, and to that woman you are very intense.

No, Patanjali doesn't mean that type of intensity. I have taken sex as an example to explain it to you because that is the only intensity that is still with you. There is no other example possible. You have become so lukewarm in your life, and exist on such a low level of energy, that there is no intensity. Somehow you manage to go to the office. Just stand on the corner of the road where people are rushing to their offices; just watch their faces – sleepy.

Where are they going? Why are they going? It seems as if they don't have anywhere else to go, so they are going to the office. They can't help it because what will they do at home? So they are going to the office, bored, automata, robotlike, going because everybody is going there and it is time to go. What do you do if you don't want to go? And holidays become such a suffering – no intensity. Coming back – look at people in the evening returning to their houses, not knowing why they are going back again, but having nowhere else to go; somehow dragging life with them. Lukewarm, a low-energy phenomenon.

That's why I have taken the example of sex – because I cannot find any other intensity in you. You don't sing, you don't dance; you don't have any intensity. You don't laugh, you don't weep. All intensity is gone. In sex, a little intensity exists; that too because of nature, not because of you.

Patanjali says ...*intense and sincere*. Religion is really like sex – deeper, higher, holier than sex, but like sex. It is one individual meeting with the whole – a deep orgasm. You melt into the whole, you completely disappear. Prayer is like love.

Yoga... In fact, the very word *yoga* means meeting, communion, meeting of the two, and such a deep and intense and sincere meeting that the two disappear. The boundaries become blurred and one exists. It cannot be in any other way. If you are not sincere and intense, bring your total being in. Only then the ultimate is possible. You have to risk yourself completely; less than that won't do.

The chances of success vary according to the degree of effort. This is one path – the path of will. Patanjali is basically concerned with the path of will, but he knows and is aware, that the other path also exists, so he gives just a footnote.

That footnote is: *Ishwara pranidhanatwa:*

Success is also attained by those who surrender to God.

Just a footnote, just to indicate that the other path is also there. Yoga is the path of will – intense effort, sincere, total. Bring your wholeness to it. But Patanjali is aware – all those who know are aware – and Patanjali is very considerate, he is a very scientific mind; he will not leave a single loophole. But that is not his path, so he simply gives a footnote just to remind you that the other path is there. *Ishwara pranidhanatwa: Success is also attained by those who surrender to God.*

With effort or surrender, the basic thing is the same: totality is needed. Paths differ, but they cannot differ absolutely. Their shape, form, direction may differ, but their inner meaning and significance has to remain the same because both lead to the divine. With effort, your totality is needed. With surrender, again your totality is needed. So to me there is only one path, and that is: bring your totality.

Whether you bring it through effort – yoga – it is up to you; or you bring it through *samarpan* – surrender, let-go – it is up to you. But always remember that totality will be needed; you have to stake yourself completely. It is a gamble, a gamble with the unknown. Nobody can say when it will happen; nobody can predict, or give you a guarantee. You gamble. You may win, you may not win. The possibility of not winning is always there because it is a very complex phenomenon. It is not as simple as it looks. But if you go on gambling, it has to happen one day.

If you miss once, don't be depressed because even a buddha misses many times. If you miss, just get up and risk again. At some time, in some unknown manner, the whole of existence culminates to help you. At some time, and in some unknown way, you hit the target exactly at the right time when the door is open. But you have to hit many times. Just go on throwing your arrow of consciousness; don't bother about the result. It is very dark and the goal is not fixed; it goes on changing. So you go on shooting your arrow in the dark. And many times you will miss.

I tell you this so you don't become depressed. Everyone misses many times, that is how it is. But if you go on and on and on and don't get depressed, it will happen. It has always happened. That's why infinite patience is needed.

What is ...*surrender to God*? How can you surrender? How does surrender become possible? – that too becomes possible if you make a lot of effort, and go on failing. Many times you make a lot of effort, you depend on yourself; effort depends on oneself. It is willpower – the path of will. You depend on yourself. You fail again and again. You stand up, you fall down; you stand up again, and you start walking. A moment comes – when you have been failing and failing and failing – and you see that your effort is the cause because your effort has become your ego.

That is the problem on the path of will. A man who is working on the path of will – making effort, using methods, techniques, doing this and that – is bound to accumulate a

THE HEART OF YOGA

certain sense of "I am": "I am superior, special, extraordinary. I am doing this and that – austerities, fasting, *sadhana*. I have done this much."

On the path of will one has to be very, very watchful of the ego because the ego is bound to come in. If you watch the ego and don't accumulate it, there is no need to surrender – because if there is no ego there is nothing to surrender. This has to be understood very, very deeply. When you are trying to understand Patanjali this is a very fundamental thing.

If you make your effort continuously for many lives, the ego is bound to arise. You have to be very watchful. You should work, you should make every effort, but don't gather the ego. Then there is no need to surrender; you may hit the target without surrendering. There is no need because the disease doesn't exist.

If there is ego, the need arises to surrender. That's why after talking about intense, sincere, total effort, Patanjali suddenly says: *Ishwara pranidhanatwa: Success is also attained by those who surrender to God.* If you feel you are continuously failing, remember that the failure is not because of the divine. The failure is happening because of your ego – from where the arrow is being shot, the source of your being. Something is happening there – a diversion. The ego is collecting there. There is only one possibility: surrender it. You have failed with it so totally, in so many ways – you did this and that, tried to do this and that and failed and failed and failed. When the frustration becomes final and you cannot see what to do, Patanjali says, "Now surrender to God."

Patanjali is rare in this sense. He does not believe in God; he is not a God-believer. God is also a technique. Patanjali doesn't believe in any God, or that there is a God. No, he says, "God is a technique." For those who fail, this is the technique – the last. If you also fail in that, there is no way. Patanjali says, "It is not a question of whether God exists or not; that is not the point at all. The point is that God is hypothetical. Without God it will be difficult to surrender. You will ask, 'To whom?'"

So God is a hypothetical point just to help surrender. When you have surrendered you will know there is no God, but that is when you have surrendered and when you have known. For Patanjali, even God is a hypothesis to help you. It is a lie. That's why I told you that Patanjali is a sly master. It is just a help for you. Surrender is the basic thing, not God. You must note this difference because there are people who think God is the basic thing. And because there is God you surrender.

Patanjali says that because you have to surrender, posit a God. God is a posited thing. When you have surrendered you will laugh. There is no God! But one more thing: there are gods – no God – a multiplicity of gods, because whenever you surrender you become a god. So don't be confused with Patanjali's God and the Christian-Jewish God.

Patanjali says, "God is the potentiality of every being. Man is as if a seed of God – every man." And when the seed flowers, comes to a fulfillment, the seed has become a god. So every man, every being, will finally become a god. God means just the ultimate culmination, the ultimate flowering. There is no God, but there are gods – infinite gods. This is a totally different conception. If you ask Mohammedans, they will say that there is only one God. If you ask Christians, they will also say that there is only one God. But Patanjali is more scientific. He says, "God is a possibility."

Everybody is carrying that possibility within the heart. Everybody is just a seed, a potentiality to become a god. When you reach to the highest beyond where nothing exists, you become a god. Many have reached before you, many will reach – and many will still be reaching after you. Everyone becomes a god finally, because everyone is a god potentially – infinite gods. That is why it becomes difficult for Christians to understand. You call Rama, Krishna, Buddha, Mahavira a god. Even an "Osho" you call a god!

It becomes impossible for a Christian to understand. What are you doing? For them, only one God exists who has created the world; for Patanjali, nobody has created the world. Millions of gods exist, and everybody is on the path to become a god. Whether you know it or not, you carry a god within your womb. You may miss many times, but how can you miss it ultimately? If you carry it within you, some day or the other the seed is going to flower. You cannot miss it absolutely – no.

This is a totally different conception. The Christian God seems to be very dictatorial, dominating the whole of existence. Patanjali is more democratic – there is no despot, dictator, Stalin, czar sitting on the throne with his only begotten son Christ by his side and the apostles all around. This is nonsense. The whole concept is as if it has been made in the image of an emperor on the throne. No, Patanjali is absolutely democratic. He says that godliness is everybody's quality. You carry it; it is up to you to bring it to its totality. If you don't want it, that too is up to you.

Nobody is sitting as a despot on the world, nobody is forcing you or creating you. Freedom is absolute. You can sin because of freedom, you can move away because of freedom, you suffer because of freedom. When you understand this, there is no need to suffer; you can come back – that too is because of freedom. Nobody is bringing you back, there is going to be no judgment day. Nobody is there to judge you except your own being. You are the doer, and the judge, you are the criminal, and the law. You are all! You are a miniature existence.

God is the supreme ruler.

He is an individual unit of divine consciousness.

Remember:

He is an individual unit of divine consciousness.
He is untouched by the afflictions of life,
action and its result.

God is a state of consciousness. It is not a person really, but "individual," so you will have to understand the difference between personality and individuality. Personality is the periphery. As you look to others, that is your personality. You say, "Nice personality, beautiful personality, ugly personality." Your personality is the decision, it is the opinion of others about you. If you are alone on the earth, will you have a personality? – no, because who will say you are beautiful, who will say you are stupid, who will say you are a great leader of men? There is nobody to say anything about you. Others opinion will not be there, and you will not have any personality.

The word *personality* comes from the Greek word *persona*. In Greek drama the actors had to use masks; those masks were called persona. From *persona* comes the word *personality*. The face that you wear when you look at your wife and smile, that is personality – persona. You don't feel like smiling, but you have to smile. A guest visits and you welcome him; deep down you never wanted him to come and you are disturbed. "Now what to do with this man?" But you are smiling and welcoming and you say, "So glad…"

Personality is that which you pose – a face, a mask. But if there is nobody in your bathroom, you don't have any personality unless you look in the mirror. Immediately the personality comes in because you start doing the work of the other opinion. You look at the face and say, "Beautiful." Now you are divided, now you are two, giving an opinion about yourself. But in the bathroom, when nobody is there and you are completely unafraid that anyone is looking through the keyhole… Because if somebody looks through the keyhole, personality comes in, you start behaving.

Only in the bathroom do you drop the personality. That's why the bathroom is so refreshing! You step out of the bath feeling so beautiful, fresh, no personality; you become an individual. Individuality is that which you are; personality is that which you show you are.

Personality is your face; individuality is your being.

In Patanjali's conception, God has no personality. He is an individual unit.

If you grow, by and by the opinions of others become childish. You don't bother about them; what they say is meaningless. It is not what they say that carries meaning; it is you, what you are, that carries the meaning. Not that they say, "You are beautiful" – this is useless. If you *are* beautiful, that is the point; what they say is irrelevant. What you are, the real, the authentic you – that is the individual.

When you drop personalities you become a sannyasin. When you renounce personalities you become a sannyasin. You become an individual unit. Now you live through your authentic center. You don't pose. When you don't pose, you are not worried. When you don't pose, you are unaffected by what others say. When you don't pose, you remain detached.

Personality cannot remain detached. It is a very fragile thing; it exists between you and the other, and it depends on the other. He can change his mind, and destroy you completely. You look at a woman and she smiles, and you feel so beautiful because of her smile. If she simply turns to you with hatred in her eyes, you are simply crushed. In fact, you are crushed because your personality has been thrown under her shoes. She walked over you; she didn't even look. Every moment you are afraid that somebody may crush your personality. Then the whole world becomes an anxiety.

A god has an individuality, but no personality. Whatever he is, that's what he shows. Whatever he is inside, is outside. In fact, in and out have disappeared for him. *God is the supreme...* In English it is translated as: *God is the supreme ruler.* That's why I say that there exists a misunderstanding about Patanjali. He calls him *purush-vishesh* in Sanskrit – a supreme being, not a ruler. I would like to translate God as the supreme. *He is an individual unit of divine consciousness.* Individual, remember, not universal, because Patanjali says that every individual is a god.

He is untouched by the afflictions of life, action and its result. Why? – because the more individual you become, the more life takes a different quality. A new dimension opens – the dimension of play. You are concerned with the personality and the outer, the crust, the periphery. Your dimension of life is that of work: worried about the result, worried about whether you will attain the goal or not, worried whether things are going to help you or not; what will happen tomorrow. A man whose life has become a play is not worried about tomorrow because he exists only today.

Jesus says, "Look at the lilies; they are so beautiful." For them, life is not work. Look at rivers, look at stars. Except man everything is beautiful and holy because the whole of existence is a play. Nobody is worried about the result. Is a tree worried whether flowers will come or not? Is a river worried whether she will reach to the ocean or not? Except man there is no worry. Why is man worried? – because he looks at life as work, not as play; the whole of existence is a play.

Patanjali says: "When one becomes centered into oneself, one becomes a player; one plays." Life is a game and it is beautiful; no need to worry about the result. The result doesn't matter, it is simply irrelevant. The thing which you are doing has value in itself. I am talking to you, you are listening to me. But you are listening with a purpose, and I am talking purposelessly. You are listening with purpose because through listening you are going to attain something – some knowledge, clues, techniques, methods, understanding – then you are going to work them out. You are wanting a result. I am talking to you purposelessly; I simply enjoy.

People ask me, "Why do you go on talking every day?" I enjoy it. It is just like birds singing – what is the purpose? Ask the rose why it goes on flowering – what's the purpose? I am talking to you because sharing myself with you is in itself a value, it has an intrinsic value. I am not looking at a result; I am not worried whether you are transformed through it or not. There is no worry. If you listen to me, that's all. If you are not worried, this very moment transformation can happen.

You are worried about how to use whatever I say and what to do about it. You are already in the future. You are not here, you are not playing the game. You are in a workshop. You are not playing the game; you are thinking how to gain some results out of it, and I am absolutely purposeless. It is how I share myself with you. I am talking, not to do something in the future; I am talking because right now, through this sharing, something is happening – and that's enough.

Remember the words *intrinsic value*, and make your every act an act of intrinsic value. Don't bother about the result because the moment you think about it, whatever you are doing becomes the means, and the end is in the future. Make the means themselves the end, make the path the goal. Make this very moment the ultimate; there is nothing beyond it. This is the state of "god"; whenever you are playing, you have some glimpses of it.

Children play, and you cannot find anything more divine than children playing. Hence, Jesus says, "Unless you become like children you will not enter the kingdom of my God." Become like children. The meaning is not to become childish because to be childish is a totally different thing; to be like children is a totally different thing. Childishness has to be dropped. That is juvenile, foolish. To be like children has to be increased. That is innocence, purposeless innocence. Profit brings the poison in; the result poisons you, and innocence is lost. *God is the supreme ruler. He is an individual unit of divine consciousness. He is untouched by the afflictions of life, action and its result.*

You can become a god right now because you are already that – just it has to be realized. You are already the case. It is not that you have to grow into a god. You have to realize that you are already that. This happens through surrender. Patanjali says, "You believe in a God, you trust in a God there, somewhere high in the universe, at the top, and you surrender. That God is just a prop to help surrender. When the surrender happens, you become a god because surrender means: 'Now I am not concerned with the results, I am not concerned with the future – I am not concerned with myself at all. I surrender.'"

When you say, "I surrender," what is surrendered? – I, the ego. Without the ego how can you think about purpose, result? Who will think about it? You are in a let-go and you go wherever it leads. Now the whole will decide; you have surrendered your decision. Patanjali says there are two ways. "Make effort total. If you don't accumulate ego, that total effort will become a surrender in itself. If you accumulate ego, then there is a way: surrender to God."

In God the seed is developed to its highest extent.

You are the seed and God is the manifestation. You are the seed and God is the actuality. You are the potential, he is the actual – God is your destiny, and for many lives you carry your destiny without looking at it because your eyes are fixed somewhere in the future. They don't look at the present. Herenow, if you are ready to look everything is as it should be. Nothing is needed. No doing is needed. Existence is perfect every single moment. It has never been imperfect, it cannot be.

If it were imperfect, how will it become perfect? Who will make it perfect? Existence is perfect; nothing at all is needed to be done. If you understand this, surrender is enough. Nothing is needed, no effort, no *pranayama*, no *bhasrika*, no *shirshasan*, no yoga postures, no meditation – if you understand that existence is perfect as it is. Look in, look out – everything is so perfect that nothing can be done except celebration.

A man who surrenders starts celebrating.

Enough for today.

4

Patanjali Is a Great Persuader

The first question:

Osho,
Please explain how a seed can flower without the bit in
between.

The seed can flower without the gap, and without the time gap in between because the seed is already flowering. You are already that which you can become. If it was not so, the seed could not flower right now; time would be needed. Then Zen is not possible; only Patanjali is the way. If you are to become something, a time process will be a must. But this is the point to understand: all those who have known have also known that "becoming" is a dream. You are already the being. You are perfect as you are.

Imperfection appears because you are fast asleep. The flower is already flowering, only your eyes are closed. If the seed has to reach to the flower, much time will be needed. And this is no ordinary flower – godliness has to flower in you. Even eternity will not be enough, it is almost impossible. If you have to flower, it is almost impossible. It is not going to happen, it cannot happen. Eternity will be needed.

No, that is not the thing. It can happen right now, this very moment; not even a single moment has to be lost. The question is not of the seed becoming a flower, the question is of opening the eyes. You can open your eyes right now and find that the flower has always been flowering. It was never otherwise, it could not have been otherwise.

Godliness is always there within you; just a look and it is manifested. Not that it was hidden in a seed; you were not looking at it. So only this much is needed – that you look at it. Whatever you are, look at it, become aware of it. Don't move like a sleepwalker.

That's why it is related that many Zen masters, when they became awakened, roared with laughter. Their disciples, their fellow travelers could not understand what had happened. Why were they roaring madly with laughter? – they were laughing because of the whole absurdity of it. They had been seeking that which was already achieved. They were running after something which was already there within them. They were seeking somewhere else for something which was hidden in the seeker himself.

The seeker is the sought; the traveler is the goal. You are not to reach somewhere else, you are to reach only yourself. This can happen in a single moment; even a fraction of a moment is enough. If the seed has to become a flower, eternity is not enough because it is a flower of God. If you are already the god, just a look back, just a look within and it can happen.

So why Patanjali? – Patanjali is needed because of you. You take such a long time to come out of your sleep, and such a long time to come out of your dreams. You are so involved in your dreams, and have so much invested in them – that's why time is needed. Time is needed not because the seed has to become a flower; time is needed because you cannot open your eyes. You have become so accustomed to having closed eyes, it has become a deeply ingrained habit. Not only that, you have completely forgotten that you are living with closed eyes. You have completely forgotten it. You think to yourself, "You are talking nonsense! My eyes are already open." And your eyes are closed.

If I say, "Come out of your dreams," you say, "I am already awake" – and this too is a dream. You can dream that you are awake, you can dream that your eyes are open; then much time will be needed – not that the flower wasn't already flowering, but it was so difficult for you to awake. There are many investments, and they have to be understood. The ego is the basic involvement. If you open your eyes you disappear; opening the eyes looks like death. It is. So you talk about it, you listen, you think about it, but you never open your eyes because if you really do open your eyes, you know that you will disappear. And then who will you be? – a nobody! A nothingness! This nothingness is there if you open your eyes; so it is better to believe that your eyes are already open, and you remain somebody.

The ego is the first involvement. The ego can exist only while you are asleep, just like dreams can exist only while you are asleep. The ego can exist only while you are asleep – metaphysically asleep, existentially asleep. Open your eyes! First you disappear, and God appears – this is the problem. You are afraid that you may disappear. But that is the door, so you listen, you think about it, but you go on postponing – tomorrow, tomorrow and tomorrow.

That's why Patanjali is needed. Patanjali says, "There is no need to open your eyes immediately; there are many steps." You can come out of your sleep in steps, in degrees. Certain things can be done today, certain things tomorrow, and the day after tomorrow… It is going to take a long time. Patanjali appeals because he gives you time to sleep. He says that there is no need to come out of your sleep right now – just a turning-over will do. Have a little more sleep, and do something else. By and by, in degrees…

Patanjali is a great persuader. He persuades you out of your sleep. Zen shocks you out of your sleep. That's why a Zen master

PATANJALI IS A GREAT PERSUADER

can hit you on your head; not a Patanjali. A Zen master can throw you out of the window; not a Patanjali. A Zen master uses shock treatment – you can be shocked out of sleep, so why go on trying to persuade you? Why waste time?

Patanjali brings you out by and by, by and by. He brings you out and you are not even aware of what he is doing. He is just like a mother. He does just the opposite, but just like a mother. A mother persuades a child to fall asleep. She may sing a lullaby to let the child feel she is there, that there is no need to be afraid. Repeating the same line again and again, the child feels seduced into sleep. He falls asleep holding his mother's hand, and feeling that there is no need to be worried. His mother is there singing, and it is beautiful. She is not saying, "Go to sleep," because that will disturb the child. She is simply indirectly persuading him. By and by, she will take her hand away and cover the child with a blanket and leave the room, and the child is fast asleep.

Patanjali does just the same in the reverse order. By and by, he brings you out of your sleep. That's why time is needed; otherwise the flower is already flowering. Look, it is already there! Open your eyes and it is there; open the door and he is standing there waiting for you. He has always been standing there. It depends on you. If you like shock treatment, Zen is the path. If you like a very gradual process, Yoga is the path. Choose! In choosing you are also very deceptive. You say to me, "How can I choose?" That too is a trick. Everything is plain. If you need time, choose Patanjali. If you are afraid of shocks, choose Patanjali. But choose! Otherwise non-choosing will become the postponement. You will say, "It is difficult to choose and unless I choose, how can I move?"

A shock treatment is immediate; it brings you down to earth immediately. My own methods are a shock treatment, they are not gradual. With me, you can hope to attain in this life; with Patanjali many lives will be needed. With me, you can also hope to attain right now, but you have many things to do before you attain.

You know the ego will disappear, you know sex will disappear.

There is no possibility of sex once you attain; it becomes absurd, silly. So you think, "A little longer... What is wrong in waiting? Let me enjoy a little longer." Anger and violence will not be possible; jealousy, possessiveness, manipulation – they will all disappear.

Suddenly you feel, "If all these disappear, what will I be then?" You are nothing but a combination of all these, a bundle of all these, and if all these disappear, only nothingness is left. That nothingness scares you. It looks like an abyss. You would like to close your eyes and dream a little longer; just like in the morning when you wake up, you would like to turn over just for five more minutes and do a little more dreaming – it was so beautiful.

One night Mulla Nasruddin woke his wife up and said to her, "Bring my specs immediately. I was having such a beautiful dream and more is promised."

Desires go on promising – more is always promised – and they say, "Do this and that, and why be in a hurry when enlightenment is always possible? You can attain anytime; there is no hurry. You can postpone it. It is a question of eternity, a concern of eternity; so why not enjoy this moment?"

You are not enjoying, but the mind says, "Why not enjoy this moment?" You have never enjoyed because a man without inner understanding cannot enjoy anything. He simply suffers, and everything becomes a suffering to him. Love – he suffers even a thing like love. The most beautiful phenomenon possible to a man asleep is love, but he suffers even through that. There is nothing better possible when you are asleep. Love is the greatest possibility, but you suffer even from that. It is not a question of love or something else – sleep is suffering, so whatever happens you will suffer. Sleep turns every dream into a nightmare. It starts beautifully, but something somewhere always goes wrong. In the end you reach hell.

Every desire leads to hell. They say that every road leads to Rome – I don't know, but I am certain of one thing: every desire leads to hell. In the beginning, desire gives you so much hope, dreams – that is the trick. That's how you are trapped. If from the very beginning desire says, "Be alert, I am leading you to hell," you won't follow it. Desire promises you heaven, and promises you, "Just a few steps and you will reach it; just come with me." It allures you, hypnotizes you and promises you many things, and being in suffering you think, "What is wrong in trying? Let us try a little of this desire also."

That too will lead you to hell because desire as such is a path to hell. Hence, Buddha says, "Unless you become desireless you cannot be blissful." Desire is suffering, desire is a dream and it exists only when you are asleep. When you are awake and alert, desires cannot befool you. You see through them, and everything is so clear that you cannot be fooled. How can money befool you and say that you will be very, very happy when you have money? Look at rich people, they are also in hell – maybe a rich hell, but it makes no difference. A richer hell is going to be worse than a poor hell. Now they have attained money and they are simply in a state of constant nervousness.

Mulla Nasruddin accumulated much wealth. He was then admitted to a hospital because he couldn't sleep and was nervous, constantly trembling and afraid – afraid of nothing in particular. A poor man is afraid of something in particular, a rich man is simply afraid. If you are afraid of something in particular, something can be done. But he was simply afraid – he didn't know why, because he had everything; there was no need to be afraid, but he was simply afraid and trembling.

He was admitted to hospital and a few things were brought to him for breakfast. One of those few things was a bowl of quivering jelly. He said, "No. I cannot eat this."

The doctor asked, "Why are you so adamant about it?"

He replied, "I cannot eat anything more nervous than me."

But a rich man is nervous. What is the nervousness and the fear about? Why is he so scared? His every desire is fulfilled and still the frustration remains. Now he cannot even dream because he has been through all the dreams, and they led nowhere. He cannot dream and he cannot gather the courage to open his eyes because there are involvements. He has promised many things in his sleep.

One night, when Buddha was about to disappear from his palace, he had wanted to tell his wife that he was going. He wanted to touch his child who had been born just a day before because he would not be back again. He went to the very door of the room. He looked at his wife – she was so fast asleep, she must have been dreaming. Her face was beautiful, smiling with the child in her arms. He waited for a few seconds at the door, and turned away. He wanted to speak to her, but he was afraid. If he said something to her, she was bound to cry and weep and create a scene.

He was also afraid of himself because if she started weeping and crying, he may become aware of his own promises: "I will love you forever and ever, and I will be with you forever and ever." And what about his child who is only one day old? She will of course bring the child to him and say, "Look what you have done to me. Why did we give birth to this child? Who will be his father now? Am I alone responsible for him? – and you are escaping like a coward." All these thoughts came to him because everybody promises in sleep. Everyone goes on giving promises, not knowing how he can fulfill them. It happens in sleep because nobody is conscious of what is happening.

Suddenly, he became aware that these things would be brought up when the family gathered together – his father and everyone else – and he is the only son and his father would be looking

PATANJALI IS A GREAT PERSUADER

at him, and in his sleep he had also promised him. He simply escaped, he simply escaped like a thief.

When he returned after twelve years, his wife asked him what had been the first thing that had come into his mind the night he left. She asked, "Why didn't you tell me? The first thing I would like to ask you – for these past twelve years I have been waiting for you – why didn't you tell me? What type of love is this? You simply left me. You are a coward."

Buddha listened silently. His wife was silent and he replied: "All these thoughts had come to me. I came to the door, I even opened it and I looked at you. In sleep I had promised many things. But if I am going to awaken, if I am going to get out of sleep, then I cannot keep the promises that I have given in sleep, and if I try to keep the promises I cannot awaken.

"So you are right. You may think I am a coward. You may think that I escaped from the palace like a thief, not like a warrior, nor like a man of courage. But I tell you now, the case is the exact opposite. At that time when I escaped, that was the moment of greatest bravery because my whole being was saying, 'This is not good. Don't be a coward.' If I had stopped, and had listened to my sleepy being, there would have been no possibility for me to awaken.

"And now I come to you; now I can fulfill something because only a man who is enlightened can fulfill. How can a man who is ignorant, fulfill anything? Now I come to you. If I had stopped that moment happening I wouldn't have been able to give you anything, but now I bring a great treasure with me, and now I can give it to you. Don't weep, don't cry; open your eyes and look at me. I am not the same man who left that night. A totally different being has come to your door. I am not your husband. You may be my wife because that is your attitude. Look at me – I am a totally different person. Now I bring treasures for you. I can make you also aware and enlightened."

The wife listened. The same problem always comes to everybody.

She started thinking about the child. If she becomes a sannyasin and moves with this beggar – her ex-husband, who is now a beggar – if she moves with him, what will happen to the child? She did not say anything, but Buddha said, "I know what you are thinking because I have passed that period where promises given in the sleepy state all crowd together and say, 'What are you doing? – your child...' You are thinking, 'Maybe wait until the child becomes a little older, until he marries; he can take over the palace and the kingdom' – and then you will follow. But remember, there is no future, no tomorrow. Either you follow me right now or you don't follow me at all."

A feminine mind is more asleep than a male mind. There are reasons for it. A woman is a greater dreamer, she lives more in hopes and dreams. She has to be a greater sleeper, otherwise it will be difficult for nature to use her as a mother. A woman must be in a deep hypnotic state, only then can she carry a child for nine months in the womb and suffer; give birth and suffer, and bring up this child and suffer. One day, the child simply leaves her and goes to another woman – and she suffers. It is such a long suffering, a woman is bound to be a greater sleeper than man. Otherwise how can you suffer so much? And she always hopes. She hopes with another child, and another – her whole life is wasted.

So Buddha said, "I know what you are thinking and I know you are a greater dreamer than me. But now I have come to cut all the roots of your sleep. Bring the child. Where is my son? Bring him."

The feminine mind played a trick again. She brought Rahul, who was twelve years old now, and said, "This is your father. Look at him – he has become a beggar! Ask him what your heritage is, what he can give you. This is your father; he is a coward! He escaped like a thief, not even telling me, and left a one-day-old child. Ask him about your heritage!"

Buddha laughed and said to Ananda, "Bring my begging

bowl." He gave the begging bowl to Rahul, and said, "This is my heritage; I make you a beggar. You are initiated, become a sannyasin." And he said to his wife, "I cut the very root, now there is no need to dream. You also awaken because this was the root. Rahul is already a sannyasin; you also awaken. Yashodhara, awaken and become a sannyasin."

The moment always comes when you are in the transit period from where sleep turns into awakening. The whole past will hold you back, and the past is powerful. The future is powerless for a sleepy man. For a man who is not sleepy, the future is powerful. For a man who is fast asleep, the past is powerful because a man who is fast asleep knows only the dreams that he has dreamed in the past. He is not aware of any future. Even if he thinks about the future, it is nothing but the past reflected again; it is just the past projected again. Only a man who is aware becomes aware of the future. The past is nothing.

Keep it in your mind. You may not be able to understand right now, but you may someday. For a sleepy man, cause is more powerful than the effect; the seed is more powerful than the flower. For a man who is awake, effect is more powerful than the cause; the flower is more powerful than the seed. The logic of sleep is: the cause produces the effect, the seed produces the flower. The logic of awakening is just the reverse: it is the flower that produces the seed, it is effect that produces the cause. It is the future that produces the past, not the past that produces the future. But for a sleepy mind, the past, the dead, the gone, is more powerful. It is not.

The yet-to-be is more powerful; the yet-to-be-born is more powerful because life is there. The past has no life; how can it be powerful? The past is already the graveyard. Life has already moved away from there; that's why it is past. Life has left it. But for you, graveyards are very powerful. For a man of awakening, the yet-to-be, the yet-to-be-born, the fresh, that which is going to happen, becomes more powerful. The past cannot hold him back.

The past holds you back. You always think about your past commitments; you always linger around the graveyard. Again and again you visit the graveyard and pay your respects to the dead. Always pay your respects to the yet-to-be-born, because life is there.

"Please explain how a seed can flower without the bit in between." Yes, it can flower because it is already flowering. The flower creates the seed, not the seed the flower. It is the flower that is going to be, that has created the whole seed. It is for you to remember: only an opening is needed. Open the doors, the sun is there waiting for you. Life is not, in fact, a progress in reality. It appears like a progress in sleep.

The being is already there. Everything is already perfect as it is – absolute, ecstatic. Nothing can be added, there is no way to improve upon it. So what is needed? – only one thing, that you become conscious and see it. This can happen in two ways: either you can be shocked out of your sleep – that is Zen; or you can be brought, persuaded, out of your sleep – that is Yoga. Choose! Just don't hang in between.

The second question:

Osho,
Is surrender to Ishwara, God, and surrender to the guru
the same?

Surrender doesn't depend on the object, it is a quality that you bring into your being. To whom you surrender is irrelevant. Any object will do. You can surrender to a tree, a river, you can surrender to anything – to your wife, your husband, your child. The problem is not there in the object; any object will do. The problem is to surrender.

It happens because of surrendering, not because of whom you have surrendered to. This is the most beautiful thing to understand: whomsoever you surrender to, that object becomes God. There is no question of surrendering to God. Where will you find God to surrender to? You will never find him. Surrender! To whomsoever you surrender, God is there. The child, husband, wife, guru becomes God; even a stone can become God.

People have even attained through stones because it is not at all a question of what you surrender to. You surrender, that opens the door and brings the whole thing with it. Surrendering, and the effort to surrender, brings an opening for you. And if you are open to a stone, you become open to the whole of existence because it is only a question of opening. How can you be open to a stone, and not be open to a tree? Once you know the opening, once you enjoy the euphoria that it brings, the ecstasy that happens just by opening to a stone... You cannot find such a foolish man who would immediately close to the remaining existence. When even opening to a stone gives you such an ecstatic experience, why not open to all?

In the beginning one surrenders to something, and then one is surrendered to all. That is the meaning of surrendering to a master. In the very experience of surrendering you have gained a clue; now you can surrender to all. The master becomes just a passage to be passed through. He becomes a door and through that door you can look at the whole sky. Remember, you cannot find God in order to surrender to, but many people think that way; they are very tricky people. They think, "When God is there, we will surrender." Now this is impossible because God is there only if you surrender. Surrender makes anything God. Surrender gives you the eyes, and everything that is brought to these eyes becomes divine. Divinity, divineness, is a quality given by surrendering.

In India, Christians, Jews and Mohammedans laugh about Hindus because they may be found worshipping a tree or a stone – not even a carved stone, not even a statue. They find a stone by the side of the road and immediately make a god out of it. No artist is needed because surrender is the art. Not even a carved, or valuable stone is needed, not even marble; any ordinary discarded stone, lying by the side of the road because it cannot be sold in the market. Hindus can immediately make a god out of it. If you can surrender, it becomes divine. The eyes of surrender cannot find anything other than the divine.

People laughed, they couldn't understand it. They thought that those people were stone worshippers, idol worshippers. They are not! Hindus have been misunderstood. They are not idol worshippers; they have found a key and the key is that you can make anything divine if you surrender. If you don't surrender, you can go on searching for God for millions of lives. You will never meet him because you don't have the quality which meets, which can meet, which can find. So the question is of a subjective surrender, not of the object to whom to surrender.

Of course there are problems. You cannot suddenly surrender to a stone because your mind goes on saying, "This is just a stone. What are you doing?" And if the mind goes on saying, "This is a stone, what are you doing?" you cannot surrender because it needs your totality.

Hence the significance of a master. A master means somebody who is standing on the boundary – the boundary of the human and the divine. One who has been a human being like you, but is no longer like you – something else has happened – one who is a plus, a human being plus. So if you look at his past, he is just like you, but if you look to his present and the future, you look to the plus. He is the divine.

It is difficult to surrender to a stone, to a river – very, very difficult. Even to surrender to a master is so difficult. So surrendering to a stone is bound to be very difficult because whenever you see a master, your mind says, "This is a human being like me, so why surrender to him?" Your mind cannot see the present, the mind can see only the past – that this man is born like you, he eats and sleeps like you, so why surrender to him? He is just like you.

He is, and yet he is not. He is both Jesus and Christ: Jesus the man, the son of man, and Christ the plus point. If you watch only the visible, he is the stone; you cannot surrender. If you love, if you become intimate; if you allow his presence to go deep in you, if you can find a rapport – that is the word, *rapport* – with his being, suddenly you become aware of the plus. He is more than human. In some unknown way he has something that you do not have. In some invisible way he has penetrated beyond the boundary of the human. You can feel this only if there is a rapport.

That is what Patanjali says: "*Shraddha*, trust, creates rapport. Rapport is an inner harmony of the two invisibles; love is a rapport. You simply fit with somebody, as if you both were born for each other. You call it love. In a moment, even at first sight, somebody simply fits with you as if you were created together and were separated, and now you have met again.

All over the world in the old mythologies it is said that man and woman were created together. In Indian mythology they have a very beautiful myth. The myth is that in the very beginning a wife and husband were created as twins, brother and sister. They were born together – as twins, wife and husband, fitting together in one womb. There was a rapport from the very beginning. From the first moment there was a rapport. They were in the womb together, holding each other – that is rapport. Then, due to some misfortune, that phenomenon disappeared from the earth.

The myth still says that there is a relationship between a man and a woman. The man may be born here, the woman may be born somewhere in Africa, or America, but there is a rapport, and unless they find each other there will be difficulties. And it is very difficult for them to find each other. The world is so vast, and you don't know where to seek and where to find. If it happens, it happens by accident.

Now scientists also believe that sooner or later we will be able to judge rapport by scientific instruments. So before a couple get married, they can go to a lab to find out whether their bioenergy fits or not. If it doesn't fit, they are in an illusion. They may think that they will be very happy together, but they cannot be because their inner bioenergy does not fit.

So you may like the nose of a woman and she may like your eyes, but that is not the point. Liking the eyes won't help, liking the nose won't help because after two days nobody looks at the nose and nobody looks at the eyes. The problem is of bioenergy – the inner energies meeting and mixing with each other; otherwise they will repel. It is just like when you have a blood transfusion: either your body accepts or rejects it because there are different types of blood. If it is the same type, the body will accept it, otherwise it simply rejects.

The same happens in a marriage. If the bioenergy accepts, it accepts; there is no conscious way to know it. Love is very fallacious because love is always focused on something. You hear the voice of a woman and it sounds good, you are allured. But that is not the point; it is a partial thing. The whole must fit. Your bioenergies should accept each other so totally that deep down you become one person. This is rapport. It rarely happens in love – so how to find it? It is still difficult. Just falling in love is not a sure criterion. Out of one thousand, nine hundred and ninety-nine times it fails. Love has proved a failure.

An even greater rapport happens with a master. It is greater than love. It is *shraddha*, trust. Not only your bioenergy meets and fits but your very soul fits. That's why, whenever someone becomes a disciple, the whole world thinks he is mad because the whole world cannot see the point. Why are you going mad about this man? You cannot explain it because it cannot be explained. You may not even be consciously aware of what has happened, but with a man, suddenly, you are in trust. Suddenly something meets, becomes one. That is rapport.

It is difficult to have that rapport with a stone. It is even difficult to have that rapport with a living master, so how can you have it with a stone? But if it happens, the master immediately becomes a god. For the disciple, the master is always a god. He may not be a god for others; that is not the point. But for a disciple, he is God, and through him the doors of divineness open. Now you have the key – this inner rapport is the key, this surrender. You can try it – you can surrender to a river.

You must have read Hermann Hesse's *Siddhartha*. He learns many things from the river which you cannot learn from a buddha; just watching the river – so many moods of the river. He became a ferryboat man, just watching the thousands of different climates around it. Sometimes the river was happy and dancing, and sometimes very, very sad, as if not moving at all; sometimes very angry and roaring against the whole of existence, and sometimes so calm and peaceful like a buddha. Siddhartha was simply a ferryman – living near the river, crossing it, watching it with nothing else to do. It becomes a deep meditation and a rapport for him, and through the river and the "riverness" of it he attains; he attains the same glimpse as Heraclitus. You can step in the same river… And you cannot. The river is the same and not the same. It is a flow, and through the river and the rapport with it, he comes to know the whole of existence as a river – a "riverness."

It can happen with anything. The basic thing to remember is surrendering.

"Is surrender to Ishwara, God, and surrender to a guru the same?" Yes. Surrender is always the same. It is just up to you to whom you are able to surrender. Find the man, seek the river and surrender. It is a risk – the greatest risk possible. That's why it is so difficult to surrender – it is a risk! You are moving in unknown territory and you are giving so much power to a man or to something you are surrendering to.

If you surrender to me, you are giving me total power. My yes is your yes, my no is your no. Even in the day if I say that it is night, you say, "Yes, it is night." You are giving total power to somebody. The ego resists. The mind says, "This is not good. Keep control. Who knows where this man will lead you? Who knows, he may say, 'Jump from the hilltop,' and then you will be dead. Who knows, this man may manipulate you, control you, exploit you." The mind will bring up all these things. It is a risk, and the mind is taking all the security measures possible.

The mind is saying, "Be watchful. Watch this man a little more." If you listen to the mind, surrender is not possible. The mind is right! It is a risk. But whenever you take it, it is going to be a risk. Watching won't help much. You can watch forever and may not be able to decide because the mind can never decide. The mind is confusion; it is never decisive. You have to bypass the mind someday or other, and say to it, "You wait and I will go. I will take the jump and see what happens."

What have you got to lose really? I'm always wondering what you have got that you are so afraid to lose, what exactly you are bringing when you surrender. You have nothing! You can gain out of it, but you cannot lose because you have nothing. You can profit out of it, but there is no possibility of any loss because you do not have anything to lose.

You must have heard Karl Marx's famous maxim, "Proletarians of the world unite because you have nothing to lose but your chains." That may be true, may not be true, but for a seeker, this is exactly the thing. What have you got to lose except your chains, ignorance, misery? But people become very attached to their misery – they cling to their misery as if it is a treasure. If you want to take away their misery, they create all sorts of barriers.

I have been watching these barriers and tricks which happen with thousands of people. Even if you want to take their misery away, they cling. This indicates a certain thing, that they don't have anything else; this is the only treasure that they have. They don't want it to be taken away because it is always better to have something than nothing. That is their logic; it is always better to have something – at least this misery – than to have nothing, than to be completely empty, than to be nobody.

Even if you are miserable, you are somebody. Even if you have hell within you, at least you have something. But watch this, observe this, and when you surrender, remember you have nothing else to give. A master is taking your misery, nothing else. He is not taking your life because you don't have any; he is taking only your death. He is not taking anything valuable from you because you don't have anything.

He is taking only the rubbish, the junkyard that you have collected through many lives; you are sitting on the heap of that junkyard and you think this is your kingdom.

He is not taking anything. If you are ready to give your misery to him, you will become capable of receiving his bliss. This is the surrender, and then the master becomes a god. Anything and anybody to whom you surrender becomes divine. Surrender makes divineness, surrender creates divineness. Surrender is a creative force.

The third question:

Osho,
Is a master needed after satori?

Yes! Even more so because satori is just a glimpse, and a glimpse is dangerous because now you enter the territory of the unknown. Before it, a master is not necessary. Before it, you were moving in the known world. Only after satori he becomes absolutely necessary because now someone is needed to hold your hand and lead you toward that which is not simply a glimpse, but becomes an absolute reality. After satori you have the taste, and the taste creates more desire. The taste becomes so magnetic that you would like to rush into it madly. Now the master is needed.

Many more things are going to happen after satori. Satori is like seeing the peak of Gourishankar, Everest, from the plains.

Some day on a clear, sunny morning, when there is no mist, you see the beautiful peak of Gourishankar rising high in the sky from thousands of miles away. This is satori. Now the actual traveling starts. Now the whole world looks useless.

This is a turning point. Now all that you knew becomes useless, all that you had becomes a burden. Now the world, the life that you had lived up to now, simply disappears like a dream because the greater has happened. This is satori, a glimpse. Soon the mist will return, and the peak will not be visible. The clouds will come, and the peak will disappear. Now you will be in an absolute uncertain state of consciousness.

The first thing will be whether what you have seen was real or just a dream because where is it now? It has disappeared. It was just a breakthrough, a gap, and you are back – thrown into your own world.

Suspicions will arise – whatever you saw, was it true? Was it really there or did you dream or imagine it? And there are possibilities. Many people do imagine it, so their suspicions are not wrong. You will imagine it many times, and be unable to make the distinction between what is real and what is unreal. Only a master can say, "Yes, don't worry. It was real," or, "Drop it! Throw it away! It was just imaginary."

Only one who has known the peak – not from the plains – who has attained the peak, and become the peak himself, only he can tell you because he has the criterion, the touchstone. He can say, "Throw it away! It's all rubbish! It is just your imagination," – because when seekers go on thinking about these things, the mind starts dreaming.

Many people come to me. Only one percent of them have the real thing; ninety-nine percent bring unreal things. But it is difficult for them to decide – impossible, not just difficult, they cannot decide.

Suddenly you feel an upsurge of energy in your backbone, in the spine. How will you decide if it is real or unreal? You have been thinking about it too much, and you have also been desiring it. Unconsciously you are sowing the seeds that it should happen, that the kundalini should rise. You have been reading Patanjali, and talking about it; then you meet some people who say that their kundalini has risen. Your ego comes in and everything is mixed… One day, suddenly you feel the upsurge; it is nothing but a creation of your mind just to satisfy you: "Don't worry – don't worry so much. Look! Your kundalini has arisen." It is just the mind imagining. Who will decide? How will you decide? You don't know the true. Only truth can become the criterion to decide whether this is true or untrue.

A master is needed even more after the first satori. There are three satoris. The first one is just a glimpse. This is even possible sometimes through drugs; this is possible through many other things – for instance, accidents. At some time or other you were climbing a tree and you fell, it was such a shock that the mind stopped for a single moment and the glimpse was there; you felt so euphoric that you were taken out of your body. You have known something.

Within a second you are back and the mind starts functioning, it was simply a shock. It is possible through an electric shock, an insulin shock, and through drugs. Sometimes even through illness it happens; you are so weak that the mind cannot function, and suddenly you have a glimpse. Through sex it is possible. In orgasm, when the whole body vibrates, it is possible.

The first glimpse is not necessarily through religious effort. That's why LSD, mescaline, or marijuana have become so important and appealing. The first glimpse is possible, and you can be caught because of it being like a drug. It can become a permanent trip, and it is very dangerous because glimpses won't help. They can help, but there is not necessarily help coming from them. They can help only around a master because he will say, "Now don't go after the glimpse. You've got the glimpse, now start traveling to reach the peak." And it isn't only to reach the peak; finally one has to become the peak.

These are the three stages: first the glimpse – it is possible through many ways, not necessarily religious. Even an atheist can have the glimpse, and a person who is not interested in religion can have the glimpse. Drugs, chemicals can give you the glimpse. Even after an operation, when you are coming round from the effects of the anesthetic, you can have the glimpse. Or while the anesthetic is being given to you and you are going under deeper and deeper, you can have the glimpse.

Many people have attained the first satori; that is not very significant. It can be used as a step for the second. The second satori is to reach the peak. That never happens accidentally. That happens only through methods, techniques, schools because it is a long effort to reach the second satori.

The third satori, Patanjali calls *samadhi*; the third is to become the peak. You can come down from the second. When you reach the peak, it may be unbearable. Sometimes bliss is unbearable – not only pain, bliss also. It is too much; one comes back to the plains.

To live on a high peak is difficult – very difficult – and one would like to come back. Unless you become the peak itself, unless the experiencer becomes the experience, it can be lost. Up to the third – *samadhi* – a master is needed. Only when the final *samadhi*, the ultimate has happened, a master is not needed.

The last question:

Osho,
While listening to you, many times certain words go very deep and there is a sudden clarity and understanding. This seems to happen only when I am attentive to the words spoken by you. But the peace that descends while listening without any particular attention to your words is equally blissful; then the words and their meaning get lost. Please give a guide to

the art of listening to you, as it is one of your best
meditations.

Don't be bothered much by words and their meaning. If you
pay too much attention, it becomes an intellectual thing. Of
course, sometimes you attain clarity. Suddenly, the clouds disappear and the sun comes out, but these will be only momentary
things and the clarity won't help much – in the next moment it is
gone. Intellectual clarity is not of much use.

If you listen to the words and their meaning you may understand many things, but you will not understand me and you will
not understand yourself either. Those things are not worthwhile
– don't bother about words and meanings. Listen to me as if I
am not a speaker but a singer, as if I am not talking to you in
words, but talking to you in sounds, as if I am a poet.

No need to go for the meaning – what I mean. Just listening to
me, without paying any attention to the words and their meanings,
a different quality of clarity will come to you. You will feel blissful;
that is the real clarity. You will feel happy, you will feel peaceful,
silent and calm. That is the real meaning.

I am not here to explain certain things to you, but to create a
certain quality within your being. I am not talking to explain; my
talking is a creative phenomenon. I am not trying to explain
something to you –you can do that through books, and there are
millions of other ways to understand these things. I am here to
transform you.

Listen to me – simply, innocently, without creating any worry
about words and their meanings. Drop that clarity, it is not of
much use. When you simply listen to me, transparent, the intellect
no longer being there – heart to heart, depth to depth, being to
being – the speaker disappears and the listener too. I am not here
and you are also not here. A rapport exists; the listener and the
speaker have become one. In that oneness, you will be transformed.
The meditation is to attain that oneness. Make it a meditation not

a contemplation, not a reflection. Something greater than words is communicated – something beyond meanings. The real meaning, the ultimate meaning, is transferred – something that is not in the scriptures and cannot be.

You can read Patanjali yourself. With a little effort, you will understand him. I'm not here talking to you so that you will be capable of understanding Patanjali; no, that is not the point at all. Patanjali is just an excuse, a peg. I am hanging something on him that is beyond scriptures.

If you listen to my words you will understand Patanjali; there will be a clarity. But if you listen to my sound, if you listen not to the words but to me, the real meaning will be revealed to you, and that meaning has nothing to do with Patanjali. That meaning is a transmission beyond scriptures.

Enough for today.

5

The Distinction between Need and Desire

Being beyond the limits of time,
he is the master of masters.

He is known as om.

Repeat and meditate on om.

Repeating and meditating on om brings about the
disappearance of all obstacles and an awakening of a
new consciousness.

Patanjali is talking about the phenomenon of God. God is not the creator; for Patanjali, God is the ultimate flowering of individual consciousness. Everybody is on the way to becoming a god. Not only you, but the stones, the rocks; every unit of existence is on the way to becoming a god. Some have become already, some are becoming, some will become.

God is not the creator, but the culmination, the peak, the ultimate of existence. He is not in the beginning, he is in the end. And of course, in a sense, he is also in the beginning because in the end only that can flower which from the very beginning has always been as a seed. God is the potentiality, the hidden possibility – this has to be remembered. So Patanjali has not a single God, he has infinite gods. The whole existence is full of gods.

Once you understand Patanjali's conception of God, God is not to be worshipped. You have to become one; that is the only worship. If you go on worshipping God that won't help. In fact, that is foolish. The worship, real worship, should consist in becoming a god yourself.

The whole effort should be to bring your potentiality to the point where it explodes into an actuality – where the seed is broken and that which was hidden from eternity becomes manifested. You are God unmanifested, and the effort is how to bring the unmanifested to the manifested level – how to bring it to the plane of manifestation.

Being beyond the limits of time,
he is the master of masters.

He is talking about his conception of God. When somebody becomes a flower, when somebody becomes a lotus of being, many things happen to him and many things start happening through him into existence. He becomes a great power, an infinite power, and through him, in many ways, others are helped to become gods in their own right. *Being beyond the limits of time, he is the master of masters.*

There are three types of masters. One is not exactly a master; rather a teacher. A teacher is one who teaches, and helps people to know about things without realizing them himself. Sometimes teachers can attract thousands of people. The only thing needed is that they should be good teachers. They may not have known themselves, but they can talk, argue, preach, and many people can become attracted through their talks, their preaching, and sermons. They may be fooling themselves by continuously talking about God. By and by, they may start feeling that they know.

When you talk about a thing, the greatest danger is that you may start believing that you know. In the beginning, when you start to talk, to teach… Teaching has some appeal because it is very ego-fulfilling – when somebody listens to you attentively, deep down it fulfills your ego that you know and he doesn't. You are the knower and he is ignorant.

It happened…

A priest, a great priest, was called to a madhouse to say a few words to the inmates. He was not expecting much, but he was surprised. One madman listened to him so attentively – he had never seen any man listen to him in such a way. He was bending forward, and he was taking each word into his heart. The man was not even blinking. He was so attentive – as if hypnotized.

When the priest had finished his sermon, he saw that the same man approached the superintendent and said something to him. He was curious. As soon as possible, he asked the superintendent, "What was that man saying to you? Was he saying something about my sermon?"

The superintendent replied, "Yes."

The priest asked, "Would you mind telling me what he said?"

The superintendent was a little bit reluctant, but said, "Yes: the man said, 'See? I am in and he is out!'"

A teacher is exactly in the same place, in the same boat, as you are. He is also an inmate. He has nothing more than you have – just a little more information. Information means nothing. You can accumulate – ordinary, average intelligence is needed to accumulate information. One need not be a genius, one need not be very talented – just average intelligence is enough. You can accumulate information, and go on accumulating; you can become a teacher.

A teacher is one who knows without knowing. He attracts people if he is a good talker, a good writer, has personality, has a certain charisma about him, magnetic eyes, a forceful body. By and by he becomes more and more skillful, but the people around him cannot be disciples, they remain students. Even if he pretends that he is a master, he cannot make you a disciple. At the most he can make you a student. A student is one who is in search of more information and a teacher is one who has accumulated more information. This is the first type of master – one who is not a master at all.

There is a second type of master, who has known himself. Whatever he says, he can say it like Heraclitus: "I have searched." Or like Buddha: "I have found." Heraclitus is more polite. He was talking to people who could not have understood if he would have said as Buddha did: "I have found." Buddha says, "I am the most perfect enlightened man that has ever happened." It looks egoistic but it is not, and he was talking to his disciples who could have understood that there was no ego at all.

Heraclitus was talking to people who were not disciples – just ordinary people. They would not have understood. He says politely: "I have searched," and leaves the other part – "I have found" – for your imagination. Buddha never says, "I have searched." He says, "I have found! This enlightenment has never happened before. It is utterly absolute."

One who has found is a master. He will attract disciples. Students are prohibited, they cannot go there by themselves. Even if they drift about and somehow reach him, they will leave as soon as possible because he will not help you to gather more knowledge. He will try to transform you. He will give you being, not knowledge. He will give you more being, not more knowledge. He will make you centered, and the center is somewhere near the navel, not in the head.

Whoever lives in the head is eccentric – this word is beautiful. The English word *eccentric* means off-center. Whoever lives in the head, is really mad – the head is the periphery. You can live in your feet or you can live in your head; the distance from the center is the same. The center is somewhere near the navel.

A teacher helps you to be more and more head-rooted; a master will uproot you from the head and replant you. Exactly… It is a replanting, and so much pain is bound to be there – suffering, anguish – because when you replant, the plant has to be uprooted from the soil where it has always been. Again, it has to be planted in new soil. It will take time. The old leaves will drop. The whole plant will pass through anguish, uncertainty, not knowing whether he is going to survive or not. It is a rebirth. With a teacher there is no rebirth; with a master there is a rebirth.

Socrates is right when he says, "I am a midwife." Yes, a master is a midwife – he helps you to be reborn. But that means you will have to die – only then you can be reborn. So a master is not only a midwife – Socrates says only half the thing – a master is also a murderer, a murderer plus a midwife. First he will kill you as you are, only then can the new come out of you. Out of your death, the resurrection.

A teacher never changes you. Whatever you are, whoever you are, he simply gives you more information. He adds to you; he retains the continuity. He may modify and refine you, and you may become more cultured, more polished, but you will remain the same. The base will be the same.

With a master, a discontinuity happens. Your past becomes as if it was never yours – as if it belonged to somebody else, as if you dreamed it. It was not real, it was a nightmare. So the continuity breaks – there is a gap. The old drops and the new comes, and between these two there is a gap. That gap is the problem, that gap has to be crossed. Many simply become scared in that gap and go back, they run fast and cling to their old past.

A master helps you to cross this gap, but for a teacher there is nothing like that; there is no problem. A teacher helps you to learn more; a master – the first job is to help you to unlearn, and that is the difference.

Someone asked Ramana Maharshi, "I have come very far to learn from you. Teach me."

Ramana laughed and said, "If you have come to learn, go somewhere else because here we do the unlearning. Here we don't teach. You already know too much; that is your problem. More learning and there will be more problems. We teach how to unlearn, how to unwind."

A master attracts disciples, a teacher attracts students. What is a disciple? Everything has to be understood minutely, only then will you be able to understand Patanjali. Who is a disciple? What is the difference between a student and a disciple? – a student is in search of knowledge, a disciple is in search of transformation, mutation. He is fed up with himself. He has come to a point, to a realization, "As I am, I am worthless – dust, nothing else. As I am is of no value."

He has come to attain a new birth, a new being. He is ready to pass through the cross, through the pangs of death and rebirth; hence, the word *disciple*. The word *disciple* comes from *discipline*; he is ready to pass through any discipline. Whatever the master says, he is ready to follow. Up to now and for many lives he has followed his own mind; he has reached nowhere. He has listened to his own mind and has got into more and more trouble. Now a point has come where he realizes, "Enough of this." He comes and surrenders to the master.

This is the discipline, the first step. He says, "Now I will listen to you. I have listened to enough of myself, to my mind; I have been a follower, a disciple, and it leads nowhere. I have realized this. Now you are my master." That means, "Now you are my mind. Whatever you say, I will listen. Wherever you lead, I will go. I will not question you because that question will come from my mind."

A disciple is one who has learned one thing through life – that your mind is the troublemaker, your mind is the root cause of your miseries. Your mind always says, "Somebody else is the cause of my misery, not me." A disciple is one who has learned that this is a trick, this is a trap of the mind. It always says, "Somebody else is responsible, I am not responsible." This is how it saves itself, protects, remains secure. A disciple is one who has understood that this is wrong – this is a trick of the mind.

Once you feel this whole absurdity of the mind… It leads you into desire, and desire leads you into frustration. It leads you into success, and every success becomes a failure. It attracts you toward beauty, and every beauty proves ugly. It leads you on and on; it never fulfills any promise. It gives you promises, but not even a single promise is fulfilled. It gives you doubt, and doubt becomes a worm in the heart – poisonous. It does not allow you to trust, and without trust there is no growth. When you understand this whole thing, only then can you become a disciple.

When you come to a master, symbolically you put your head to his feet. This is dropping your head; this is putting your head to his feet. Now you say, "I will remain headless. Now, whatever you say will be my life." This is the surrender. A master has disciples who are ready to die and be reborn.

And there is the third – a master of masters. A teacher of students first; a master of disciples second; a master of masters third. Patanjali says that when a master becomes a god – and to become a god means one who transcends time; for whom time does not exist, ceases to exist; for him there is no time. He is one who has come to understand the timelessness, the eternity; who has not only changed and become good, who has not only changed and become aware, but who has gone beyond time – he has become a master of masters. Now he is a god.

What will a master of masters be doing? This stage comes only when a master leaves the body – never before it. You can be aware in the body, and in the body you can realize that there is no time. But the body has a biological clock. It feels hunger and after a time gap, again hunger; satiety and hunger, sleep, disease, health. In the night the body has to go to sleep; in the morning it has to wake. The body has a biological clock. So the third master happens only when he finally leaves the body – when he will not be coming back to the body again.

Buddha has two terms. The first he calls nirvana, enlightenment. When Buddha became enlightened he remained in the body. That is enlightenment, nirvana. After forty years he left the body; he calls it the absolute nirvana – *mahaparinirvana*. He became a master of masters, and he has remained a master of masters.

Every master, when he leaves the body permanently, and to which he will not be returning, becomes a master of masters. Mohammed, Jesus, Mahavira, Buddha, Patanjali, have remained masters of masters, and they have been continuously guiding masters, not disciples.

Whenever somebody on the path of Patanjali becomes a master, immediately there is a contact with Patanjali, whose soul floats in the infinite, the individual consciousness which he calls God. Whenever a person following Patanjali's path becomes enlightened, a master, immediately there is a communication with the original master who is now a god.

Whenever somebody following Buddha becomes enlightened, a relationship immediately comes into existence. He is suddenly joined with Buddha – Buddha who is no longer in the body, Buddha who is no longer in time and no longer in space, but still is; Buddha who has become one with totality, but still is. This is very paradoxical and very difficult to understand because we cannot understand anything which is beyond time. Our whole understanding is within time; our whole understanding is within space. When somebody says that Buddha exists beyond time and space, it makes no sense to us.

When you say that Buddha exists beyond space, it means he does not exist anywhere in particular. How can somebody exist without existing anywhere in particular? He exists, simply exists! You cannot indicate where; you cannot say where he is. In that sense he is nowhere, and in that sense he is everywhere. For the mind which lives in space, it's very difficult to understand something beyond space. But whoever follows Buddha's methods and becomes a master immediately has a contact. Buddha still goes on guiding people who follow his path; Jesus still goes on guiding people who follow his path.

In Tibet there is a place on Kailash where, every year on the day Buddha left the world, the full-moon night of Vaishakh, five hundred masters gather together. And at this place, where five hundred masters gather together every year, they have a realization of Buddha descending – again becoming visible.

This is an old promise and Buddha still fulfills it. Five hundred masters have to be there – not one less, because then it will not be possible. These five hundred masters help as a weight, as an anchor, for Buddha to descend. Even one less master, and the phenomenon doesn't happen. Because sometimes it had happened that there were not five hundred masters. That year there was no contact – no visible contact. Invisible contact remains, but no visible contact.

But Tibet has many masters, so it was not difficult. Tibet is the most enlightened country; it has remained so up to now. It will not be so in the future, thanks to Mao. He has destroyed the whole subtle pattern that Tibet has created. The whole country was a monastery. Monasteries exist in other countries; Tibet existed in the monastery.

It was a rule that one person from every family had to take sannyas and become a lama. This rule was made so that at least every year five hundred masters were always available. When five hundred masters gather together on Kailash just at midnight – twelve o'clock – Buddha is again visible. He descends into time and space.

He has been guiding; every master goes on guiding. Once you are near a master, not near a teacher, you can trust. Even if you don't attain enlightenment in this life, there will be a continuous subtle guidance for you – even if you don't realize that you are being guided.

Many of Gurdjieff's people have come to me. They have to come because Gurdjieff has been throwing them toward me. There is nobody else to whom Gurdjieff can throw or push them. This is unfortunate, but it is so – that now there exists no master in Gurdjieff's system, so he cannot make contact. Many of Gurdjieff's people will be coming to me sooner or later, and they are not aware of it because they cannot understand what is happening. They think this is just accidental.

If a master exists on a certain path in time and space, the original master can go on sending instructions. That's how religions have always remained alive. Once the chain is broken, the religion becomes dead. For example, the Jaina religion has become dead because there is not a single master to whom Mahavira can go on sending new instructions. With every age things change: mind changes, techniques have to be changed, methods have to be devised, new things have to be added, old things have to be deleted. Every age needs much work.

If a master exists on a certain path, the original master who is now a god can continue. But if the master is not there on the earth, the chain is broken and the religion becomes dead. It happens many times. For example, Jesus never intended to create a new religion; he never thought about it. He was a Jew, and he was receiving direct instructions from old Jewish masters who had become gods. But Jews wouldn't listen to the new instructions. They said, "This is not written in the scriptures. What are you talking about? In the scriptures it is written that if somebody hits you with a brick, you throw a rock at him; an eye for an eye, and a life for a life." And Jesus started saying, "Love your enemy – and if he hits you on one cheek, give him the other."

It is not written in the Jewish scriptures, but this was the new instruction because the age had changed. This was a new method to work it out, and Jesus was receiving it directly from gods – gods in Patanjali's sense: the old prophets. But that was not written in the scriptures. Jews killed him not knowing what they were doing. That's what Jesus said in the last moment, when he was on the cross. "God forgive these people, because they don't know what they are doing." They are committing suicide. They are killing themselves because they are breaking the link from their own masters.

And that happened. The murder of Jesus became the greatest calamity for the Jews, and for two thousand years they have suffered because they have had no contact. They live with the scriptures; they are the most scripture-oriented people on the earth. The Talmud, the Torah – they live with the scriptures and whenever an effort is made from the higher sources beyond time and space, they don't listen.

This has happened many times. That's how new religions are born. It is unnecessary, there is no need. But the old people won't listen. They say, "Where is it written?" It is not written. It is a new instruction, a new scripture. If you don't listen to the new scripture, the new instruction will become a new religion. And see, the new religion always seems to be more powerful than the old. It has the latest instructions, and it can be more helpful to man.

Jews remained the same. Christianity spread out over half the earth; now half of the world is Christian. Jainas have remained a very small, tiny minority in India because they won't listen. They don't have any living master. They have many sadhus, monks – many, because they can afford it; they are a rich community – but not a single living master. No instructions can be given through the higher sources. This was one of the greatest revelations of Theosophy in India – in this age, all over the world – that masters continuously go on instructing. Patanjali says that this is the third category of masters: the master of masters. This is what he means by a god. *Being beyond the limits of time, he is the master of masters.*

What is time and how does one go beyond it? Try to understand. Time is desire because for desire, time is needed. Time is a creation of desire. If you have no time, how can you desire? There is no space for desire to move. Desire needs the future. That's why people who live with millions of desires are always afraid of death. Why are they afraid of death? – because death cuts time immediately. There is no longer any time and you have millions of desires, and here comes death.

Death means now there is no longer any future; death means now there is no longer any time. The clock may go on ticking, but you will not be ticking. Desire needs time to fulfill it – future. You cannot be desirous in the present; desire doesn't exist in the present. Can you desire anything in the present? How will you desire it? Because if you desire, the future has immediately entered. Tomorrow has entered, or the next moment. How can you desire in this moment, here now?

Desire is impossible without time; time is also impossible without desire. They are a phenomenon together, two aspects of the same coin. When one becomes desireless, one becomes timeless. Future stops, past stops. Only the present is there. When desire stops, it is as if a clock goes on ticking and the hands have been taken off. Just imagine, a clock goes on ticking with no hands, so you cannot say what the time is.

A man without desire is a clock ticking without hands.

That is the state of a buddha. He lives in the body; the clock goes on ticking because the body has its own biological process to continue. It will be hungry and it will ask for food. It will be thirsty and ask for a drink. It will feel sleepy and will go to sleep. The body has needs, so it is ticking. But the innermost being has no time; the clock is without hands.

But because of the body you are anchored in the world, in that world of time. Your body has a weight, and because of that weight gravitation still functions on you. When the body is left, and when a buddha leaves the body, the ticking itself stops. He is pure consciousness: no body, no hunger and no satiety; no body, no thirst – no body, then no need.

Remember these two words: *desire* and *need*. Desire is of the mind; need is of the body. Desire and need – you are a clock with hands. Only need, no desire – you are a clock without hands. When need drops, you have gone beyond time. This is eternity, and beyond time is eternity.

For example: if I don't look at the clock, I don't know what the time is – and I have to continuously look, the whole day. Even if I have looked at it five minutes before, I have to look again because I don't know exactly, because now with no time inside, only the body is ticking.

Consciousness has no time. Time is created when the consciousness desires something – immediately time is created. In existence there is no time. If man is not on the earth, time will immediately disappear. Trees tick, rocks tick. The sun will rise and the moon will set and everything will continue as it is, but there will be no time because time doesn't come with the present, it comes with the memory of the past and the imagination of the future.

A buddha has no past. He is finished with it, he doesn't carry it. A buddha has no future. He is also finished with that because he has no desire. But needs are there because the body is there. A few more karmas have to be fulfilled; the body will go on ticking for a few more days, just the old momentum will continue. You have to wind a clock. Even if you stop winding it, it will continue to tick for a few hours or a few days. The old momentum will continue. *Being beyond the limits of time, he is the master of masters.*

When both need and desire disappear, time disappears. And remember to make a distinction between desire and need, otherwise you can get into a very deep mess. Never try to drop needs. Nobody can drop them, unless the body drops. And don't get confused with what is what. Always remember what need is and what desire is. Need comes from the body and desire comes from the mind. Need is animal; desire is human. Of course, when you feel hungry you need food. If you stop when the need stops, your stomach immediately says, "Enough." But the mind says, "A little more. It is so tasty." This is desire. Your body says, "I am thirsty," but the body never asks for Coca Cola. The body says, "Thirsty" so you drink. You cannot drink more water than is needed, but you can drink more Coca Cola. It is a mind phenomenon.

Coca Cola is the only universal thing in this age – even in Soviet Russia nothing has entered, but Coca Cola has. Even the iron curtain doesn't make any difference because the human mind is the human mind.

Always watch where need stops and desire starts. Make it a continuous awareness. If you can make the distinction, you have attained something – a clue to existence. Need is beautiful, desire is ugly. But there are people who go on desiring, and they go on cutting their needs. They are foolish, stupid. You cannot find bigger idiots in the world because they are doing just the opposite.

There are people who will fast for days and desire heaven. Fasting is cutting the need and desiring heaven is helping there to be more desire. They have a greater amount of time than you because they have to think of heaven – they have a vast time, with heaven included in it. Your time stops at death. They will say to you, "You are a materialist." They are spiritualists because their time goes on and on. It covers heavens – not only one, but seven – and even *moksha*, the final liberation, is within their time limit. They have a vast amount of time, and you are materialists because your time stops at death.

Remember, it is easy to drop needs because the body is so silent you can torture it. The body is so adaptive that if you torture it too long it becomes adjusted to your torture. And it is dumb – it cannot say anything. If you fast for two or three days it will say, "I am hungry, I am hungry." But your mind is thinking of heaven, and without being hungry you cannot enter there. It is written in the scriptures, "Fast" – so you don't listen to the body. It is also written in the scriptures, "Don't listen to the body – the body is the enemy."

The body is a dumb animal; you can go on torturing… For the first few days it will say something, and if you start a long fast – at the most for the first week… On the fifth or sixth day, the body stops protesting because nobody is listening, so it starts making adjustments of its own. It has a reservoir for ninety days. Every healthy body has a reservoir of fat which will last for ninety days as an emergency – not for fasting.

It might happen that you are lost in a forest and can't get food, or maybe there is a famine; the body has a reservoir for ninety days. It will feed itself; it eats itself. It has a two-gear system. Ordinarily it asks for food. If you supply it with food, the reservoir remains intact. If you don't supply it, it goes on asking for two or three days. If you still don't supply it, it simply changes gear. The gear is changed; it starts eating itself.

That's why in fasting you lose one kilo every day. Where is this weight going? – it is disappearing because you are eating your own fat, your own flesh. You have become a man-eater, a cannibal. Fasting is cannibalism. Within ninety days you will be a skeleton, your reservoir will be finished. You will have to die.

It is easy to be violent to the body, it is so dumb. But to the mind it is difficult because the mind is so vocal, it won't listen. The real thing is to make the mind listen and cut the desires. Don't ask for heaven and paradise.

I was just reading a book about new religions in Japan. As you know, Japanese people are very technically skilled; they have created two paradises in Japan. Just to give you a glimpse, they have made a small paradise on a hill station to show you how it is up there. You just go and have a glimpse. They have made a beautiful place and have kept it absolutely clean with flowers and trees and shaded areas and beautiful small bungalows. They give you a glimpse of paradise so that you start desiring.

There is no paradise. Paradise is a creation of the mind. There is no hell. That too is a creation of the mind. Hell is nothing but missing paradise, that's all. First you create, and then you miss because it is not there. And these people, these priests, the poisoners – they always help you to desire. First they create the desire, and hell follows. Then they come to save you.

Once I was driving along a very primitive road. It was summer – and suddenly I came to a part of the road that was so muddy that I couldn't believe how it was possible. There had been no rain, but there was a patch of mud for almost half a mile. I thought it couldn't be very deep so I drove into it; I became stuck. It was not only muddy, it had many potholes. I waited to see if someone with a truck might come along and help me.

A farmer did come along with a truck. When I asked him to help me, he said that he would charge me twenty rupees. So I said, "Okay! Take twenty rupees, but just get me out of this." When I was out, I said to the farmer, "At this price you must be doing the job day and night."

He replied, "No, not at night because I have to carry the water from the river to this road. Who do you think creates this mud here? And I have to have a little sleep because business starts early in the morning."

These are the priests. First they carry water from a faraway river and create mud; you are then bogged down, and they help you. There is no paradise and no hell; no heaven, no hell. You are being exploited, and you will be exploited unless you stop desiring.

A man who doesn't desire cannot be exploited. No priest and no church can exploit him. It is because you desire that you create the possibility of being exploited. Cut your desires as much as you can because they are unnatural. Never cut your needs because they are natural; fulfill your needs.

Look at the whole thing. There are not very many needs, not many at all. And they are so simple. What do you really need? – food, water, shelter, somebody to love you or somebody that you can love. What else do you need? – love, food, shelter – simple needs. Religions are against all these needs. They are against love; they say to practice celibacy. They are against food; they say to practice fasting. They are against shelter; they say to become monks, to move, and become wanderers – homeless. They are against needs. That's why they create hell. And you suffer more and more, and become more and more in their hands. You ask for help, and the whole thing is created.

So never go against needs, but always remember to cut desires. Desires are useless. What is a desire? – it is not a desire for shelter.

Desire is always for a better shelter. Desire is comparative; need is simple. You need a shelter, desire needs a palace. Need is very, very simple. You need a woman to love, or a man to love. Desire? – desire needs a Cleopatra. Desire is simply for the impossible; need is for the possible. If the possible is fulfilled you are at ease. Even a buddha needs that.

Desires are foolish. Cut desires and become aware. And you will be beyond time. Desires create time – if you cut desires you will be beyond time. While the body is there its needs will remain, but if desires disappear, this is your last or, at the most, last but one life. Soon you will also disappear. One who has attained desirelessness will sooner or later become beyond needs because then the body is not needed. The body is a vehicle of the mind; if the mind isn't there, the body isn't needed anymore.

He is known as om.

This God, the perfect flowering, is known as om. Om is the symbol of the universal sound. You hear thoughts, words within you, but never the sound of your being. When there is no desire, no need, when the body has dropped, when the mind disappears, what will happen? – the real sound of the universe itself is heard. That is om.

All over the world, people have realized this om.

Mohammedans, Christians, Jews – they call it amen. It is om. Zoroastrians, Parsis, call it *ahura mazda*. That *a* and *m* – *ahura* is from *a* and *mazda* is from *m* – it is *aum*. They have made it a deity.

That sound is universal. When you stop, you hear it. Right now you are talking so much, chattering within yourself, that you cannot hear it. It is a silent sound. It is so silent that unless you have completely stopped you will not be able to hear it. Hindus have called their gods a symbolic name – om. Patanjali says: *He is known as om.*

If you want to find a master, a master of masters, you will have to get more and more attuned to the sound of om.

Repeat and meditate on om.

Remember, Patanjali is so scientifically oriented that he will not leave out even a single word, and will not even use one more word.

Repeat and meditate... Wherever he says, "Repeat om," he always adds *meditate.* The difference has to be understood.

Repeat and meditate on om.

Repeating and meditating on om brings about the disappearance of all obstacles and an awakening of a new consciousness.

If you repeat and don't meditate, it will be Maharishi Mahesh Yogi's Transcendental Meditation – TM. If you repeat and don't meditate, it is a hypnotic device. You fall asleep. It is good because falling asleep is beautiful. It is healthy, and you will come out of it feeling calm. You will feel more of a well-being, more energy, more zest. But it is not meditation. It is like a tranquilizer and a pep pill together. It gives you a good sleep, and you feel very good in the morning. More energy is made available to you, but it is not meditation – it can become dangerous. If you use it for a long time, you can become addicted to it. The more you use it, the more you will realize that there comes a point where you are stuck. If you don't do it, you feel you are missing something; if you do it, nothing happens.

This point has to be remembered: whenever you are meditating, if you feel that if you don't do it you will miss it and if you do it nothing happens, then you are stuck. Immediately, something is needed to be done. It has become an addiction, just like smoking cigarettes. If you don't smoke, you feel something is missing. You continuously feel that something has to be done; you feel restless. If you smoke, nothing is gained. That is the definition of addiction. If something is gained, it is okay; however nothing is gained – it has become a habit. If you don't do it, you feel miserable; if you do it, no bliss comes out of it.

Repeat and meditate – repeat om, om, om – and stand apart from this repetition. Om, om, om; the sound is all around you and you are alert, aware, watching, witnessing. That is meditating. Create the sound within you and still remain a watcher on the hill. In the valley, the sound is moving – om, om, om – and you are standing above, watching, witnessing. If you don't watch, you will fall asleep. It will be a hypnotic sleep. Transcendental Meditation appeals to people in the West because they have lost the capacity to sleep well.

In India, nobody bothers about Maharishi Mahesh Yogi because people are so fast asleep, snoring. They don't need it. But when a country becomes rich and people are not doing physical labor, their sleep is disturbed. Either you take tranquilizers or TM. Of course, TM is better because it is not so chemical. But it is still a very, very deep hypnotic device.

Hypnosis can be used in certain cases, but should not be made a habit because ultimately it will give you a sleepy being. You will move around as if in hypnosis; you will look like a zombie. You will not be aware and alert. The sound of om is such a lullaby because it is a universal sound. If you repeat it, you can become a complete alcoholic through it, intoxicated. Then comes the danger because the real thing is not to become intoxicated. The real thing is to become more and more aware. There are two possibilities to drop out of your worries.

Psychoanalysts divide the mind into three layers: the first they call the conscious, the second they call the subconscious, the third they call the unconscious. And the fourth they don't know yet – Patanjali calls it the superconscious. If you become more alert, you move above the conscious and reach the superconscious. That is the stage of a god – superconscious, super-aware.

If you repeat a mantra without meditating, you fall into the subconscious. If you fall into the subconscious it will give you a good sleep, good health, and a feeling of well-being. But if you continue with it, you will fall into the unconscious – you have become a zombie. And this is very, very bad. It is not good.

A mantra can be used as hypnosis. If you are being operated on in a hospital it is okay. Rather than having an anesthetic, it is good to be hypnotized; it is less evil. If you don't feel sleepy, it is better to do TM than take a tranquilizer. It is less dangerous, less harmful. But it is not meditation.

So Patanjali continuously insists: *Repeat and meditate on om.* Repeat and create the sound of om all around you, but don't be lost in it. It is such a sweet sound, you will be lost. Remain alert – remain more and more alert. As the sound goes deeper, you become more and more alert; so the sound relaxes your nervous system, but not you. The sound relaxes your body, but not you. The sound sends your whole body and physical system into sleep, but not you.

A double process has started: the sound drops your body into a restful state and the awareness helps you to rise to the superconscious. The body moves to the unconscious, becomes a zombie, fast asleep, and you become a superconscious being. Your body reaches the bottom and you reach the peak. Your body becomes the valley and you become the peak. This is the point to be realized. *Repeat and meditate… Repeating and meditating on om brings about the disappearance of all obstacles and an awakening of a new consciousness.*

The new consciousness is the fourth – superconsciousness. But remember, repetition on its own is not good. Repetition is just to help you to meditate. Repetition creates the object; the most subtle object is the sound of om. If you can be aware of the most subtle, your awareness also becomes subtle.

When you watch gross things, your awareness is gross. When you watch a sexual body, your awareness becomes sexual. When you watch something that is an object of greed, your awareness becomes greed. Whatever you watch you become. Remember this – the observer becomes the observed.

Krishnamurti insists again and again: "The observer becomes the observed." Whatever you observe, you become. So if you observe the sound of om – which is the deepest sound, the deepest music, the sound without sound, the sound which is uncreated, *anahat*; the sound which is just the nature of existence – if you become aware of it, you become that, you become a universal sound. They both – subject and object – meet and merge and become one. That is the superconscious where the object and the subject have dissolved; where the knower and the known are no more. Only one remains; the object and the subject are bridged. This oneness is yoga.

The word *yoga* comes from the root *yuj*. It means meeting, combining together. It happens when the subject and the object are yoked together. The English word *yoke* also comes from *yuj*, the same root from where *yoga* comes. When the subject and the object are yoked together – sewn together so that they are no longer separate, bridged – the gap disappears. You attain a superconsciousness.

That's what Patanjali calls: *Repeating and meditating on om brings about the disappearance of all obstacles and an awakening of a new consciousness.*

Enough for today.

6

Osho:
The Beginning of a Tradition,
Not the End

The first question:

Osho,
Do you receive instructions from any master of
masters?

I am not on any ancient path, so a few things have to be understood. I am not like Mahavira, who was the end of a long series
of twenty-four *tirthankaras* – he was the twenty-fourth. In the past,
twenty-three had become masters of masters, gods, on the same
path, the same method, the same way of life, the same technique.

The first was Rishabhdeva and the last was Mahavira. Rishabhdeva had nobody in the past to look to. I am not like Mahavira,
but like Rishabhdeva. I am a beginning of a tradition, not the
end. Many more will be coming on the same path. So I cannot
look to anybody for instructions; that's not possible. A tradition
is born and it dies, just as individuals are born and die. I am the
beginning, not the end. When somebody is in the middle of
the series or at the end, he gets instructions from the master
of masters.

The reason why I am not on any path? – I have worked with
many masters, but I have never been a disciple. I was a wanderer,

wandering through many lives, crisscrossing many traditions, being with many groups, schools, methods, but never belonging to anybody. I was received with love, but I was never a part – a guest at the most, on an overnight stay. That's why I learned so much. You cannot learn so much on one path; that's impossible. If you move on one path, you know everything about it, but nothing about anything else. Your whole being is absorbed in it. That has not been my way. I have been like a bee going from one flower to another, gathering many fragrances. That's why I can be at ease with Zen, with Jesus, Jews, Mohammedans, and with Patanjali – all diverse ways, and sometimes diametrically opposite.

But to me, a hidden harmony exists. That's why people who follow one path are unable to understand me. They are simply baffled, bewildered. They know a particular logic, a particular pattern. If the thing fits into their pattern, it is right. If it doesn't fit, it is wrong. They have a very limited criterion. To me, no criteria exist because I have been with so many patterns that I can be at ease anywhere. Nobody is alien to me and I am not a stranger to anybody. But this creates a problem. I am not a stranger to anybody, but everybody becomes a stranger to me – this has to be so.

If you belong to no particular sect, everybody thinks of you as the enemy. Hindus, Christians, Jews, Jainas, are all against me – and I am against nobody. Because they cannot find their pattern in me, they are against me.

I am not talking about a pattern, but the deeper pattern which holds all the patterns. There is a pattern, another pattern, and another pattern, millions of patterns. All the patterns are held by something underground which is the pattern of patterns – the hidden harmony. They cannot look at it, but they are not at fault. When you live with a certain tradition, a certain philosophy, a certain way of looking at things, you become attuned to it.

In a way, I was never attuned to anybody – not so much that I could have become a part of them. In a sense it is a misfortune, but in another sense it proved a blessing. Many who worked with me achieved liberation before me. It was unfortunate for me. I lagged far behind because I never worked totally with anything; I was moving from one to another.

Many of those who started with me, achieved. Even a few of those who started after me achieved before me. This was unfortunate, but in another sense this has been a blessing because I know every home. I may not belong to any home, but I am at home everywhere. That is why I have no master of masters – I was never a disciple. To be directed by a master of masters, you have to be a disciple of a certain master. Then you can be directed. You know the language. I am not directed by anybody, but helped by many. The difference has to be understood: I am not directed, I don't receive any orders such as, "Do this or don't do that," but I am helped by many.

Jainas may not feel that I belong to them, but Mahavira feels it because he at least can see the pattern of patterns. The followers of Jesus may not be able to understand me, but Jesus can. So I am helped by many. That's why many people are coming to me from different sources. At this present time you cannot find such a gathering as this anywhere on the earth. Here there are Jews, Christians, Mohammedans, Hindus, Jainas, Buddhists from all over the world. And many, many more will be coming soon; that's help from many masters. They know I can be helpful to their disciples. They will be sending many more – but with no instructions because as a disciple I never received instructions from any master. Now there is no need. Just some help, and that is better – I feel I have more freedom. Nobody can be as free as I am.

If you receive directions from Mahavira, you cannot be as free as I am. A Jaina has to remain a Jaina; he has to go on speaking against Buddhism, against Hinduism. He has to because it is a fight of many patterns and traditions. And traditions have to fight if they want to survive. They have to be argumentative for the sake of the disciples. They have to say, "That is wrong."

Only then can the disciple feel, "This is right." Looking at what is wrong, the disciple feels what is right.

You will be at a loss with me. If you are here with just your intellect you will be confused. You will go crazy because this moment I say something and the next moment I contradict it. In this moment I am talking about one tradition, and in another moment I am talking about another one. Sometimes I am not talking about any tradition; I am talking about me, and you cannot find it anywhere in any scripture.

But I am helped, and the help is beautiful because I am not supposed to follow it. I am not forced to follow it. It is up to me. The help is given unconditionally. If I feel like doing it, I do it; if I don't feel like it, I don't do it. I have no obligations to anybody.

If you become enlightened someday, then you can receive. If I am not in the body, you can receive instructions from me. When a tradition starts, this always happens to the first person. It is a beginning, a birth, you are near a birth process and it is the most beautiful when something is born because it is at its most alive. By and by, as a child grows, it is coming closer and closer to death. A tradition is at its freshest when it is born. It has a beauty of its own – incomparable, unique.

The people who listened to Rishabhdeva, the first Jaina *tirthankara*, had a different quality. When they listened to Mahavira, the tradition was thousands of years old. It was just on the verge of dying. It died with Mahavira.

When masters are no longer born in a tradition, it is dead. It means the tradition is no longer growing. The Jainas closed it. With the twenty-fourth *tirthankara* they said, "Now, no more masters, no more *tirthankaras*." And to be with Nanak was beautiful because something new was coming out of the womb – the womb of the universe. Just as you watch a child being born – a mystery, an unknown penetrating the known, the bodiless becoming embodied – it is fresh like dewdrops. Soon everything will be covered with dust. Soon, as time passes, things will become old.

By the time of the tenth guru of the Sikhs, the tenth master, things became dead. They closed the line and said, "Now, no more masters. The scripture itself will be the master." That's why they called their scripture Guru Granth, the master scripture. Now there will be no more people; just a dead scripture will be the master. When a scripture is dead it is futile – not only futile, it is poisonous. Don't allow anything dead to be in your body. It will create a poison; it will destroy your whole system.

Here, something new is born, a beginning. It is fresh, but that's why it is also very difficult to see. If you go to the Gangotri, the source of the Ganges, it is so tiny there – fresh, of course. It will never be so fresh again because when it flows it gathers many things, it accumulates and becomes more and more dirty. It is at its dirtiest at Kashi, but you call it the Holy Ganges because it is so vast. It has accumulated so much, that now even a blind man can see it. At the Gangotri – at the beginning, at the source – you need to be very perceptive. Only then can you see; otherwise it is just trickling drops of water. You can't believe that even this trickling is going to become the Ganges – unbelievable.

Right now, it is difficult to see what is happening because it is a very, very tiny stream, just like a child. People missed with Rishabhdeva, the first Jaina *tirthankara*, but they could recognize Mahavira – see? Jainas don't think much of the first, Rishabhdeva. In fact, their whole homage is paid to Mahavira. To the Western mind, Mahavira is the originator of Jainism. And because they pay so much respect to Mahavira in India, how can anyone feel that somebody else was the originator? Rishabhdeva has become legendary, forgotten; he may have been, may not have been, and he doesn't seem to be historical. He is from the hoary past, and you don't know much about him. Mahavira is historical; he is like the Ganges near Varanasi, Kashi – so vast.

Remember that the beginning is small, but never again will the mystery be so deep as in the beginning. The beginning is life and the end is death. With Mahavira, death enters the Jaina tradition. With Rishabhdeva, life entered, came down from the Himalayas above to the earth.

I have nobody to be responsible to and nobody to get instructions from, but much help is available. If you take it in its totality, it is more than any single master can instruct. When I am talking about Patanjali, he is helpful. I can talk exactly as if he was talking here. In fact, I am not talking; these are not commentaries. It is he himself using me as a vehicle. When I am talking about Heraclitus, he is there – but as a help. You have to understand this, and become more perceptive so that you can see the beginning.

To move into a tradition when it has become a great force does not take much perceptivity, or sensitivity. To come just when things are beginning, in the morning, is difficult. By the evening many have come, but they have come because the thing has become so vast and powerful. In the morning only a chosen few come; those who have the sensitivity to feel that something great is being born. You cannot prove it right now; time will prove it. It will take thousands of years to prove what was being born, but you are fortunate to be here. And don't miss the opportunity, because this is the freshest point and the most mysterious.

If you can feel it, if you can allow it to go deep into you, many things will become possible in a very short period of time. It is not yet respectable to be with me, it is not prestigious. In fact, only gamblers can be with me – those who do not bother or worry about what others say. Respectable people cannot come here. By and by, after a few years, when the tradition becomes dead, it becomes respectable. Then people will come. But they will be dead people; they will come only when something becomes respectable. They will come because of the ego.

You are not here because of the ego; with me there is nothing to gain, for the ego at least. You will lose. With Rishabhdeva, only people who were alive and courageous, daring and adventurous moved with him; with Mahavira, dead businessmen – not gamblers. That is why Jainas have become a business community. The whole community is based on business; they don't do anything except that. And business is the least courageous thing in the world. That's why businessmen become cowards. They were cowards in the first place; that's why they became businessmen.

A farmer is more courageous because he lives with the unknown; he doesn't know what is going to happen, whether the rains will come or not – nobody knows. And how can you believe in clouds? You can believe in banks, but you cannot believe in clouds. Nobody knows what is going to happen; he hangs there with the unknown. But he lives a more courageous life – one of a warrior.

Mahavira was a warrior, and all the twenty-four Jaina *tirthankaras* were warriors. So what was the unfortunate thing that happened? What happened to make all of Mahavira's followers become businessmen? It happened because they came to be with him only when the tradition was glorious; when it had a legendary past, and had already become a myth and was respectable to be involved with.

Dead people come only when something becomes dead; alive people come only when something is alive. And many, many younger people will be coming to me. Even if an older person comes to me, he is bound to be younger in his heart. Old people look for prestige, respect; they go to dead churches and temples where there is nothing but emptiness and a past. What is the past? – an emptiness. Anything alive is herenow, anything alive has a future because the future grows out of it. The moment you start looking at the past there can be no growth.

You say: "Do you receive instructions from any master of masters?" No! But I receive help, which is more beautiful. I have been a loner, a vagabond with no home, passing through, learning, moving, never staying anywhere. So I have nobody to look up to. If I had to find something, I had to find it myself. Much help was available, but I had to work it out. In a way that is going to be a great help because I don't depend on any code.

I watch the disciple. There is nobody for me to look to as a master. I have to look at the disciple more deeply to find the clue which will help him. I have to look into you. That's why my teaching, my methods, differ with each disciple. I have no universal formula, I cannot have; no fixed rules – I have to respond. I do not have a readymade discipline. Rather, it is a growing phenomenon; every disciple adds to it. When I start working with a new disciple I have to look into him, seek, find what will help him, how he can grow. And each time, with each disciple, a new code is born.

You are going to be really in a mess when I am gone because there will be so many stories from each disciple, and you will not be able to make any head nor tail of it – because I am talking to each individual as an individual. The system is growing through him, and is growing in many, many directions. It is a vast tree, with many branches, many sub-branches, pointing in all directions.

I don't receive any instructions from the masters, I receive instructions from you. When I look into you, in your unconscious, in your depth, I receive instructions from there and I work it out for you. It is always a new response.

The second question:

Osho,
Why do masters need directions from a master of
masters? Are they not enough unto themselves when
they have reached enlightenment? Or are there stages
of enlightenment too?

No, in fact there aren't stages, but when a master is in the body, and when he leaves the body and becomes bodiless, there is a difference – not exactly stages. It is just like if you are standing under a tree by the side of the road, and you can see a patch of the road, but cannot see beyond that patch. Then you climb the tree. You remain the same; nothing is happening to you or your consciousness, but you have climbed the tree, and from the top you can see for miles right around from one side to the other.

You can take a flight in an airplane – nothing happens to you; your consciousness remains the same, but now you can see for thousands of miles. In the body you are on the road – by the side of the road – encased in the body. The body is the lowest point in existence because it means it is still committed to matter, still being with matter. Matter is the lowest point and God is the highest point.

When a master attains enlightenment in the body, the body has to fulfill its karmas, the past *samskaras*, past conditionings. Every account has to be closed; only then can the body be left. It is like this: your airplane has arrived, but you have a lot of businesses to finish up. All the creditors are there, and they are asking you to close your accounts before you leave. There are many creditors because for many lives you have been promising, doing things, acting, behaving; sometimes good, sometimes bad, sometimes a sinner, sometimes a saint. You have accumulated so much. Before you leave, the whole of existence demands that you complete everything.

When you become enlightened, you know that you are not the body, but you owe many things to the body and the material world. Time is needed. Buddha and Mahavira lived for forty years after their enlightenment in order to pay for everything they owed, and to complete every circle that they had started. There is no new action, but the old things hanging around have to be finished, the old hangover has to be finished. When all the accounts are closed, now you can catch your plane.

Up to now, with matter, you have been moving horizontally – just like in a bullock cart. Now you can move vertically. Now you can go upward. Before this, you have always been going forward or backward; there was no vertical movement. The higher you rise... The God, the master of masters, is the highest point from where there is total perception. Your consciousness is the same; nothing has changed. An enlightened man has the same consciousness as the supreme state of consciousness, God – no difference of consciousness. But the field of perception is different; now he can look everywhere.

In the time of Buddha and Mahavira there was a great debate. It will be useful to understand it at this point for this question. There was a debate. The followers of Mahavira used to say that Mahavira is omnipotent, omniscient, omnipresent, *sarvagya*, all-knowing.

In a way they are right because once you are freed from matter and the body, you are God. But in a way they are wrong because you may be freed from the body, but you have not yet left it. The identification is broken; you know that you are not the body, but still you are in it. It is as if you live in a house, and suddenly you find out that it doesn't belong to you; it is somebody else's house and you were living in it.

But there again, to leave the house you will have to make arrangements, you will have to remove things. It will take time. You know the house isn't yours, your attitude has changed. Now you are not worried about the house – whatever happens to it. If on the next day it falls down and becomes a ruin, it doesn't matter to you. If you leave and the next day it catches fire, it doesn't matter to you; it belongs to somebody else. Just a moment before you were identified with the house; it was yours. If there had been a fire, or if the house had fallen down, you would have been very worried. Now the identification is not there.

Mahavira's followers are right in a sense because when you have come to know yourself you have become all-knowing. But Buddha's followers used to say that this is not right – a buddha can know if he wants to know something, but he is not all-knowing. They used to say that if Buddha wants to, he can focus his attention in any direction, and wherever he focuses his attention he will be able to know. He is capable of omniscience, but not omniscient. The difference is subtle, delicate, but beautiful. They said if he knows everything and all things constantly, he will go mad. The body cannot bear that much.

They are also right. A buddha in the body can know anything if he wants to. His consciousness, because of the body, is like a torch – you use the torch in the dark. You can come to know anything if you focus; light is with you. But a torch is a torch; it is not a flame. A flame will give light in all directions; a torch focuses in a particular direction – wherever you want it to. The torch has no choice. You can look to the north, and it will reveal the north. You can look to the south, and it will reveal the south. But all four directions are not revealed together. If you move the torch to the south, the north is closed. It is a narrow flow of light.

This was Buddha's followers' standpoint. Mahavira's followers used to say that he is not like a torch, he is like a lamp – all directions are revealed. But I favor Buddha's followers' standpoint. When the body is there, you are narrowed down. The body is a narrowing. You become like a torch – because you cannot see from the hands, you can see only from the eyes. If you can see only from the eyes, you cannot see from your back, because you don't have any eyes there. You have to move your head.

With the body, everything is focused and narrow. The consciousness is unfocused and flowing in all directions, but the vehicle, the body, is not flowing in all directions; it is always focused – so your consciousness becomes narrowed down to it. But when the body is no longer there, when a buddha has left the body, there is no problem. All directions are revealed together.

That's the point to be understood; that's why even an enlightened person can be guided because an enlightened person is still tethered to the body, anchored in the body, in the narrow body. And a god is unanchored, floating in the highest sky. From there he can see all directions. From there he can see the past, future, present. From there his view is unclouded. That's why he can help.

Even if you become enlightened in the body, your view is clouded. The body is there all around you. The status of consciousness is the same, the innermost reality of the consciousness is the same, the quality of the light is the same. But one light is tethered to the body and has become narrow; one light is not tethered to anything at all – just a floating light. Guidance is possible in the highest of skies.

"Why do masters need directions from a master of masters?" – that's the reason. "Are they not enough in themselves when they have reached enlightenment or are there stages of enlightenment too?" They are enough. They are enough to guide disciples; they are enough to help disciples. Nothing is needed, but still they are tethered, and one who is untethered is always a good help. You cannot look in all directions, but he can.

You can also move and look, but that has to be done. This is what I am doing; having no instructor above, nobody to guide me, I have to be continuously on the move – looking from this and that direction, watching from this and that direction, looking at you through many standpoints so that your totality can be seen. I can see through, but I have to move around you. Just a glance will not be helpful because a glance will be narrowed through the body. I have a torch and I am moving all around you, looking from every standpoint possible.

In a way it is difficult because I have to work more. In a way it is very beautiful because I have to work more and I have to look from every standpoint possible. And I come to know many things which ready-made instructions cannot do. When the master of masters in Patanjali's ideology – a god – gives instructions, he gives no explanations; he simply gives instructions. He simply says, "Do this; don't do that."

To those who follow these instructions, they will look like they are ready-made. It is bound to be so because they say, "Do this," and give no explanation. Very coded instructions are given. Explanations are very difficult – there is also no need for them because when it is given from a higher standpoint it is okay. One just has to be obedient.

The master is obedient to the master of masters, and you have to be obedient to the master. An obedience follows. It is just like a military hierarchy – not much freedom. Not much is allowed. Order is order. If you ask for explanations, you are rebellious. This is the problem, one of the greatest problems humanity has to face now; man cannot now be obedient as in the past. You cannot simply say, "Don't do this." An explanation is needed – and not any ordinary explanation will do. An authentic explanation is needed because the very mind of humanity is no longer obedient. Now rebelliousness is built in; a child is now born rebellious.

It was totally different in the days of Buddha and Mahavira. Now everybody is taught to be individual, to stand on his own, to believe in himself. Trust has become difficult. Obedience is not possible. If somebody follows without questioning, you think he is a blind follower. He is condemned. Now only a master who has all the explanations can help you – more than you require, and who can exhaust you completely. You go on asking; he can go on answering you. A moment comes when you are tired of asking, and you say, "Okay, I will follow."

It was never like this. Before, it was simple; when Mahavira said, "Do this," you did it. But now this is not possible, simply because man is so different. The modern mind is rebellious, you cannot change it. This is how it has come to be through evolution, and nothing is wrong in it. And that is why old masters are falling by the way; nobody listens to them anymore. You go to see them, they have instructions, beautiful instructions, but they don't provide any explanation. Now, the first thing is the explanation. The instruction should follow as a syllogism. All explanations should be given first, and then the master should say, "Therefore, do this."

It is a lengthy process, but it's how it is. Nothing can be done. And in a sense it is a beautiful growth because when you simply trust, your trust has no salt in it, no tension in it. Your trust has no sharpness in it. It is a hodgepodge – shapeless, no tonality, no color in it. It is just gray. But when you can doubt, argue, reason, and a master can satisfy all of these, there arises a trust which has a beauty of its own because it has been achieved against the background of doubt.

It has been achieved against all doubts, it has been achieved against all challenges. It has been a fight. It was not simple and cheap; it has been costly. When you achieve something after a long fight, it has a meaning of its own. If you simply pick it up on the road – it was just lying there – and take it home, it has no beauty. If there are Kohinoors all over the earth, who will bother about taking them home? If a Kohinoor is just an ordinary pebble lying anywhere, who will bother about it?

In the old days, faith was like pebbles all over the earth; now it has to be a Kohinoor, now it has to be a precious achievement. Instructions won't help. A master has to be so deep in his explanations that he exhausts you. I never say to you, "Don't ask." In fact, the case is just the opposite. I say to you, "Ask! And you don't find questions!"

I will bring all the questions possible from your unconscious to the surface, and I will solve them. Nobody can say to you that you are a blind follower. I will not give you a single instruction without totally satisfying your reason – no, because that is not going to help you in any way.

Instructions are given from the masters of masters, but they are just quoted words – sutras: "Do this; don't do that." In the new age, that won't help. Man is now so rational that even if you are teaching irrationality you have to reason about it. That's what I am doing: teaching you the absurdity, the irrational, teaching you the mysterious – and through reason. Your reason has to be used so much that you become aware that it is futile – and throw it away. You have to be spoken to about your reason so much that you get fed up with it; you drop it on your own, not through

THE HEART OF YOGA

an instruction – because instruction can be given, but you will cling to it. And that won't help.

I'm not going to say to you, "Just trust me." I'm creating the whole situation in which you cannot do otherwise. You will have to trust. It will take some time, a little longer than simple obedience, but it is worth it.

The third question:

Osho,
We, in our unawareness and egoistic state, are not
always in touch with the master. But is the master
always in touch with us?

Yes, because a master is in touch with all the four layers of you. Your conscious layer is only one of the four layers. But it is possible only when you have surrendered and accepted him as your master – not before that. If you are just a student, learning, when you are in touch, the master is in touch; when you are not in touch, he is also not in touch.

This phenomenon has to be understood. You have four minds. The first, the supermind is the possibility of the future, of which you carry only seeds – nothing has sprouted, only seeds, just the potentiality. Then there is the conscious mind – a very small fragment with which you reason, think, decide, argue, doubt, believe. This conscious mind is in touch with a master to whom you have not surrendered; so whenever this is in touch, the master is in touch. If this is not in touch, the master is not in touch. You are a student, and you have not taken the master as a master. You still think of him as a teacher. Teacher and student exist in the conscious mind. Nothing can be done because you are not open; all three of your doors are closed. The superconscious is just a seed, and you cannot open its doors.

The subconscious is just below the conscious. That is possible

if you love. If you are here with me only because of your reasoning, your conscious door is open. Whenever you open it, I am
there. If you don't open it, I am outside and cannot enter. Just
below the conscious is the subconscious. If you are in love with
me – not just in a teacher–student relationship, but in a more
intimate, lovelike phenomenon – your subconscious door is
open. Many times the conscious door will be closed by you. You
will argue against me; sometimes you will be negative, sometimes
you will be against me. But that doesn't matter. The unconscious
door of love is open and I can always remain in touch with you.

But that too is not a perfect door because sometimes you can
hate me. If you hate me, you have also closed that door. Love is
there, but the opposite, hate, is also there – it always is with love.
The second door will be more open than the first – because the
first changes its moods so fast that you don't know; every moment
it goes on changing. Just one moment before it was here, the next
moment it is not here; it is a momentary phenomenon.

Love is a little longer. It also changes its moods, but they have
longer periods. Sometimes you will hate me. In thirty days there
will be almost eight days, one week or more, when you will hate
me. But for three weeks it is open. With reason, a week is too
long; it is an eternity. With reason, one moment you are here
with me, another moment you are against me; for, against – it
goes on. If the second door is open and you are in love with me,
even if the door of reason is closed, I can remain in contact.

The third door is below the subconscious, and that is the
unconscious. Reason opens the first door – if you feel convinced
by me. Love opens the second door, which is bigger than the
first; if you are in love with me – not convinced, but in love –
feeling an affinity, a harmony, an affection.

The third door opens by surrender. If you are initiated by me,
if you have taken the jump into sannyas, if you have taken a
jump and said to me, "Now – now you be my mind. Take my
reins and I will follow." Not that you will always be able to do it,

but just the very gesture that you have surrendered opens the third door. The third door remains open. You may be against me rationally. It doesn't matter; I am in touch. You may hate me, it doesn't matter; I am in touch – because the third door always remains open. You have surrendered. It is very difficult to close the third door – very, very difficult. It is difficult to open, it is difficult to close. It is difficult to open, but not as difficult as it is to close it. But that too can be closed because you have opened it; that too can be closed. You can decide someday to take your surrender back. Or, you can go and surrender to somebody else. But that never – almost never – happens because with these three doors the master is working to open the fourth door.

So the possibility that you will take your surrender back is almost impossible. Before you have taken it back, he must have opened the fourth door which is beyond you. You cannot open it, you cannot close it. The door that you open, you remain the master to also close it. The fourth door has nothing to do with you. That is the superconscious. These three doors need to be open so the master can forge a key for the fourth door. And you don't have the key, otherwise you could open it yourself. The master has to forge it; it is forged because the owner himself doesn't have the key.

The whole effort of a master is to have enough time from opening these three doors to enter the fourth, forge a key and open it. Once it is opened, you are no more. You cannot do anything now. You may close the first three doors – he has the key to the fourth and is always in contact. Even if you die, it doesn't matter. You can go to the very end of the earth, to the moon, it doesn't make any difference – he has the key to the fourth. In fact, a real master never keeps the key. He simply opens the fourth and throws the key in the ocean. So there is no possibility of stealing it or doing anything – nothing at all.

I have forged a fourth door key for many of you and have thrown it away, so don't trouble yourself unnecessarily; it is futile, now nothing can be done. Once the fourth is opened, there's no problem. All the problems existed before this because at the very last moment the master was getting the key ready, and the key is difficult.

For millions of lives the door has remained closed; it has gathered all sorts of rust. It looks like a wall, not like a door. It is difficult to find where the lock is – and everybody has a separate lock, so there is no master key. One key for all won't help because everyone is as individual as your thumbprint. Nobody else has that print anywhere – not in the past, and never in the future. Your thumbprint is simply yours, a single phenomenon. It is never repeated.

Your inner lock is also like your thumbprint – absolutely individual – no master key can help. That's why a master is needed because a master key cannot be purchased. Otherwise, once a key is made, everyone's door can be opened. No, everyone has a separate type of door, a separate type of lock, his own locking system. You have to watch, find and forge a key, a special key for it.

Once your fourth door is open, the master is in constant touch with you. You may forget him completely – it makes no difference. You may not remember him – it makes no difference. The master leaves the body – it makes no difference. Wherever he is, wherever you are, the door is open. And this door exists beyond time and space. That's why it is the supermind; it is the superconscious.

You say: "We in our unawareness and our egoistic state are not always in touch with the master, but is the master always in touch with us?" – yes, but only when the fourth door is opened. With the third door, he is more or less in contact. With the second door, half the time he is almost in contact. With the first door, he is only momentarily in contact.

So allow me to open your fourth door – and the fourth door is opened in a certain moment. That moment is when all three of your doors are open. Even if a single door is closed, the fourth cannot be opened. It is a mathematical puzzle. This condition is needed: your first, conscious door is open, and your second door is open – your subconscious, your love; you have surrendered, and have taken a step into initiation – your third, unconscious door is open.

In a certain moment when all three doors are open, the fourth can be opened. While you are awake, the fourth is difficult to open. While you are asleep, only then... So my real work is not in the day, it is in the night when you are fast asleep snoring because then you don't create any trouble. You are so fast asleep, you don't reason against it. You have forgotten about reasoning. Your heart functions well in deep sleep. You are more loving than when you are awake because when you are awake many fears surround you, and because of those fears love is not possible. When you are fast asleep, those fears disappear and love flowers. Love is a night flower.

You must have seen the flower, Queen of the Night – it flowers in the night. Love is a night queen, it flowers in the night – because of you; there is no other reason. It can flower in the day, but then you have to change yourself. Tremendous change is needed before love can flower in the day.

That's why you notice that people who are intoxicated are more loving. Go into any bar where people have been drinking too much, and you will almost always find them very loving. See two drunkards walking on the street hanging onto each other – so loving – as if they were one! They are asleep.

When you aren't afraid, love flowers. Fear is the poison. When you are deep asleep you are already surrendered because sleep is a surrender. And if you have surrendered to a master, he can enter your sleep. You will not even be able to hear his footsteps. He can enter silently and work. It is a forgery, a deception, just like thieves entering in the night when you are asleep. A master is a thief. When you are fast asleep and don't know what is happening, he enters you and opens the fourth.

Once the fourth is opened, there is no problem. Every effort and trouble that you can create, happens only before the fourth is open. The fourth is a point of no return. Once the fourth is open, the master can be with you twenty-four hours – there is no problem.

The last question:

Osho,
How can one cut desires without suppressing them?

Desires are dreams, they are not realities. You cannot fulfill them and you cannot suppress them because to fulfill a certain thing it needs to be real; to suppress a certain thing it also needs to be real. Needs can be fulfilled and they can be suppressed. Desires can neither be fulfilled nor can they be suppressed. Try to understand this because it is very complex.

A desire is a dream; if you understand this it disappears, and then there is no need to suppress it. What is the need to suppress a desire? For example: you want to become very famous. This is a dream, a desire because the body doesn't bother if it is famous or not. In fact, when you become famous, the body suffers very much. You don't know how the body suffers when a person becomes famous. There is no peace. You are continuously bothered, troubled by others because you are so famous.

Somewhere Voltaire has written, "When I was not famous, I used to pray to God every night, 'Make me famous. I am nobody, so make me somebody.' Then I became famous. I started to pray, 'Enough is enough; now make me nobody again' – because before, when I used to go onto the streets of Paris, nobody would look at me and I felt so sad. Nobody would pay any attention to me. It was as if I didn't exist at all. I would go into different restaurants and come out; nobody, not even the waiters, would pay any attention to me."

And what about kings? – they didn't know Voltaire existed. He writes: "Then I became famous. It became difficult to walk about on the streets because people would gather around me. It was difficult to go anywhere. Even to go into a restaurant and have a relaxed meal, a crowd would gather around."

A time came when it was almost impossible for him to get out of his house, because in those days there was a superstition in Paris, that if you could get a piece of cloth from a very famous man and make a locket out of it, it brought you good luck. So wherever he went he would come back naked because people would tear his clothes – and they would also harm his body. Police were needed to escort him, whenever he left or returned to Paris.

So he used to pray, "I was wrong. Simply make me nobody again because I can't go and watch the river, or the sunrise, or go to the hills, I cannot move. I have become a prisoner."

Famous people are always prisoners. The body doesn't need to be famous; it is absolutely okay, it doesn't need such nonsense. It needs simple things – food; it needs water, a shelter when it is too hot – its needs are very, very simple. The world is mad because of desires, not because of needs. And people go mad. They go on cutting down on their needs and growing and increasing their desires. There are people who would like to drop one meal a day, but they cannot drop their newspaper, they cannot drop going to the cinema or smoking. But they can drop food – needs can be dropped, desires cannot. The mind has become a despot.

The body is always beautiful; remember it. This is one of the basic rules I give you – a rule unconditionally, absolutely, categorically true: the body is always beautiful, the mind is ugly. It is not the body that has to be changed. There is nothing in it that needs to be changed. It is the mind. The mind means desiring. The body needs, but the body's needs are real needs.

If you want to live, you need food. Fame is not needed to live; respect is not needed to be alive. You need not be a very great man or a very great painter – famous, known to the whole world. You need not be a Nobel Prize winner to live because a Nobel Prize doesn't fulfill any need of the body.

If you want to drop needs, you will have to suppress them because they are real. If you fast, you have to suppress hunger. Then there is suppression. Every suppression is wrong because it is a fight inside; you want to kill the body. The body is your anchor, your ship which will lead you to the other shore. The body keeps the treasure, the seeds of the divine within you, protected. Food, water, shelter is needed for that protection; comfort is needed for the body because the mind doesn't want any comfort.

Look at modern furniture, it is not comfortable at all, but the mind says, "This is modern, and what are you doing sitting in an old chair? The world has changed and modern furniture has come in." Modern furniture is really weird. You feel uncomfortable in it; you cannot sit in it for long – but it is modern! The mind says that the modern must exist because how can you be out-of-date? Be up-to-date!

Modern clothes are uncomfortable, but they are modern and the mind says that you have to be up with the fashion. Man has done so many ugly things because of fashion. The body needs nothing. These are the mind's needs, you cannot fulfill them – never – because they are unreal. Only unreality cannot be fulfilled. How can you fulfill an unreal need which is in fact not there? What is the need of fame? Just meditate on it. Close your eyes and look. Where is it needed in the body? How will it help if you are famous? Will you be healthier if you are famous? Will you be more silent, peaceful? What will you gain out of it?

Always make the body the criterion. Whenever the mind says something, ask the body, "What do you say?" If the body says that it is foolish, drop it – there is no suppression because it is an unreal thing. How can you suppress an unreal thing? In the morning, you get out of bed and you remember a dream. Do you suppress it or do you fulfill it? In a dream, you dreamed that you have become the emperor of the whole earth. Now what do you do? Should you try? Otherwise the question arises, "If I don't try, it is suppression." But a dream is a dream! How can you suppress a dream? A dream disappears by itself. You have only to be aware. You have to only know that it is a dream. When a dream is a dream and known as such, it disappears.

Try to find out what a desire is and what a need is. A need is body oriented; a desire has no orientation in the body. It has no roots, it is just a floating thought in the mind. And almost always your body-needs come from your body and your mind-needs come from others. Somebody purchases a beautiful car... Somebody else has purchased a beautiful car, an imported car, and now your mind-need arises. How can you tolerate this?

Mulla Nasruddin was driving and I was sitting with him. It was a very hot summer day. The moment we entered his neighborhood he immediately closed all the windows of his car.

I said, "What are you doing?"

He replied, "What do you mean? Should I let all the people in my neighborhood know that I don't have an air-conditioned car?"

He was perspiring; I was also perspiring along with him. It was like an oven, hot – but how can you allow your neighbors to know that you don't have an air-conditioned car?

This is a mind-need. The body says, "Drop it! Are you mad?" It is perspiring. It is saying, "No!" Listen to the body; don't listen to the mind. The mind's needs are created by others around you; they are foolish, stupid, idiotic. Body-needs are beautiful and simple. Fulfill your body-needs; don't suppress them. If you suppress them, you will become more and more ill and diseased. Never bother about the mind-needs, once you know that's what it is. Is there really much difficulty in knowing it? What is the difficulty? – it is so simple to know that this is a mind-need.

Simply ask the body, inquire in the body; go and find the root. Is there any root cause for it?

You will look foolish. All your kings and emperors are foolish. Just take a look; they are clowns. Dressed up with thousands of medals, they look so foolish. What are they doing? And they have suffered a long time for this. To attain this, they have passed through so many miserable times and they are still miserable. They have to be miserable. The mind is the door to hell and the door is nothing but desire. Kill desires. You will not find any blood coming out of them because they are bloodless.

But kill a need and there will be bloodshed. Kill a need and you will die in part. Kill a desire and you will not die; on the contrary, you will become freer. More freedom will come out of dropping desires. If you can become a man of need with no desires, you are already on the path and heaven is not far off.

Enough for today.

7

With the Chanting of Om,
All Obstacles Disappear

Disease, languor, doubt, carelessness, laziness,
sensuality, delusion, impotency and instability are the
obstacles that distract the mind.

Anguish, despair, tremors and irregular breathing are
the symptoms of a distracted mind.

To remove these, meditate on one principle.

Patanjali believes – and not only believes, he knows also – that sound is the basic element of existence. Just as physicists say that electricity is the basic element, yogis say that sound is the basic element. They agree with each other in a subtle way.

Physicists say that sound is nothing but a modification of electricity, and yogis say that electricity is nothing but a modification of sound. Both are true. Sound and electricity are two forms of one phenomenon, and to me that phenomenon is not known yet and will never be known. Whatever we know will be just a modification of it. You may call it electricity, you may call it sound; you may call it fire like Heraclitus, you may call it water like Lao Tzu – that depends on you. But all these are modifications – forms of the formless. That formless will always remain unknown.

How can you know the formless? Knowledge is possible only when there is a form. When something becomes visible, you can know it. How can you make invisibility the object of knowledge? The very nature of invisibility is that it cannot be objectified. You cannot pinpoint where it is, what it is. Only something visible can become the object.

So whenever anything is known, it will just be a modification of the unknown. The unknown remains unknown. It is unknowable. So it depends on you what you call it, and it depends on the

use you are going to put it to. For the yogi, electricity is not relevant. He is working in the inner lab of being. There, sound is
more relevant because through sound he can change many phe-
nomena inside, and through sound he can also change the inner
electricity. Yogis call it *prana* – the inner bioenergy or bioelec-
tricity. And through sound that can be changed immediately.
That's why, when listening to classical music, you feel a certain
silence surrounding you; your inner body energy is changed.
Listen to a madman and you will feel you are also going crazy,
because the madman's body electricity is in a chaos and his
words and sounds carry that electricity to you. Sit with an enlightened person and suddenly you feel everything within you is
falling into a rhythm, suddenly you feel a different quality of
energy arising in you.

Patanjali says, "The repetition of om and meditation on it
destroys all obstacles." What are the obstacles? Now he describes
each obstacle, and how they can be destroyed by repeating the
sound of om and meditating on it. We will have to ponder over it:

Disease, languor, doubt, carelessness, laziness,
sensuality, delusion, impotency and instability are the
obstacles that distract the mind.

Take each one. *Disease...* To Patanjali, disease means dis-ease. It
is a nonrhythmic way of your inner bioenergy. You feel uncomfortable. If this discomfort, this dis-ease, continues, sooner or later it
will affect your body. Patanjali will absolutely agree with acupuncture, and in Russia a man named Kirlian will absolutely agree with
Patanjali. Acupuncture is not concerned with enlightenment, but it
is concerned with how the body becomes diseased, how illness
happens. Acupuncture has discovered seven hundred points on the
body where the inner bioenergy touches the physical body – seven
hundred touchpoints all around the body.

When the electricity is not flowing in a circle in these seven hundred points – some gaps may appear, a few points are not functioning, the electricity is no longer moving through a few points; some blocks occur, the electricity is cut, and it is no longer a circle – then disease happens. So acupuncture believes that without any medicine, and without any other treatment, if you allow the bioenergy flow to become a circle, the disease disappears. Acupuncture was born five thousand years ago, almost the same time when Patanjali was alive.

As I told you, after two thousand five hundred years there comes a peak of human consciousness. It happened in the time of Buddha; in China with Lao Tzu, Chuang Tzu, Confucius; in India with Buddha, Mahavira and others; in Greece with Heraclitus; in Iran with Zarathustra. The peak phenomenon happened. All the religions that you see now in the world derive from that moment of human consciousness. All the rivers of all the religions have been flowing from that peak, the Himalaya, for these two thousand five hundred years.

In just the same way, two thousand five hundred years before Buddha, there was a peak phenomenon. There was Patanjali, Rishabhdeva – the originator of Jainism; the Vedas, the Upanishads, acupuncture in China, Yoga in India and Tantra – these all happened. They attained a peak. Never again has that peak been surpassed. From that very remote past, five thousand years ago, Yoga, Tantra and acupuncture have been flowing like rivers.

There is a certain phenomenon which Jung has called synchronicity. When a certain principle is born, not only one person, but many people on the earth become aware of it; it is as if the whole earth is ready to receive it. Einstein is reported to have said, "If I had not discovered the theory of relativity, then within a year somebody else would have discovered it." Why? – because many people all over the earth were working in the same direction.

When Darwin discovered the theory of evolution – that man has evolved out of monkeys, that there is a constant struggle for the survival of the fittest – another man, Wallace Russell, also discovered it. He was in the Philippines, and they were friends. But for many years they hadn't known each other. Darwin was working continuously for twenty years, but he was a lazy man. He had many fragments and everything was ready, but he would not make a book out of it and he would not present it to the scientific society of those days.

Again and again his friends would advise him, "Do it – otherwise someone else will." And one day a letter arrived from the Philippines and the whole theory was presented by Russell in that letter. He was a friend, but they were working separately. They never knew that they were both working on the same theory. Darwin became afraid; what was he to do? Russell would become the discoverer, when he himself had known the principle for twenty years. He rushed, and somehow managed to write a report, and presented it to the scientific society.

After three months, everyone else became aware that Russell had also discovered it. Russell was really a very beautiful person. He declared that the discovery should go to Darwin because for twenty years, whether he had presented it or not, he was the discoverer.

This happens many times; suddenly a thought becomes very prominent, as if it is trying to take a womb somewhere. This is the way of nature, it never takes risks. One man may miss, so many men have to be tried. Nature never takes risks! A tree will drop millions of seeds. One seed may miss, may not fall on the right ground, may be destroyed, but with millions of seeds it's not possible that all the seeds will be destroyed.

When you make love, millions of seeds are released by the man in one ejaculation. One of them will reach the egg of the woman – but there are millions. In one ejaculation, a man releases almost as many seeds as there are men on the earth right now. One man, in one ejaculation, can give birth to the whole earth, to the whole population of the earth. Nature takes no risks. It tries many ways. One may miss, two may miss, a million may miss, but with millions at least one will reach and become alive.

Jung discovered a principle which he calls synchronicity. It is a rare thing. We know one principle – of cause and effect. A cause produces an effect. Synchronicity says that whenever something happens, many similar things happen parallel to it. We don't yet know why it happens because it is not a cause and effect phenomenon. They are not related with each other as cause and effect.

How can you relate Buddha and Heraclitus? But the same principle. Buddha had never heard of Heraclitus, Heraclitus we cannot imagine ever knew about Buddha. They lived in separate worlds. There was no communication. But both gave the same principle of flow, of riverlike existence, of momentary existence to the world. They are not causing each other, they are parallel. A synchronicity exists as if the whole existence at that moment wants to produce a certain principle and wants to make it manifest – its manifestation will not depend only on Buddha or Heraclitus; it will try many. There were others also, who went into oblivion; they were not so prominent. Buddha and Heraclitus became the most prominent. They were the most forceful masters.

In the days of Patanjali, a principle was born. You can call it the principle of *prana* – bioenergy. In China it took the form of acupuncture, in India it took the form of the whole system of Yoga. Why do you feel discomfort when the body energy is not flowing rightly? – a gap exists in you, an absence, and you feel something is missing. This is dis-ease in the beginning. First it will be felt in the mind, first it will be felt in the unconscious as I told you.

You may not be aware of it, but it will come first in your dreams. In your dreams you will see illness, disease, somebody dying, something wrong. A nightmare will happen in your unconscious because the unconscious is nearest to the body and nearest to nature. From the unconscious it will come up to the subconscious, and you will feel irritated. You will feel that the stars are wrong, as whatever you do goes wrong. You would like to love a person, you try, but you cannot. You would like to help someone, but you only hinder. Everything goes wrong.

You think that it is some bad influence, from some star high in the sky. No, it is something in the subconscious, some discomfort – you get irritated, angry, and the cause is somewhere in the unconscious. You find the cause somewhere else. Then the cause comes to the conscious, and you start feeling that you are ill, and it moves to the body. It has always been moving to the body, and suddenly you feel ill.

In Russia a photographer, Kirlian, a rare scientist, has discovered that six months before a person becomes ill, that illness can be photographed. And this is going to be one of the greatest discoveries in the world of the twentieth century. It will transform the whole concept of man, disease, medicine, everything. It is a revolutionary concept, and he has been working at it for thirty years. He has almost proved everything scientifically – that when a disease comes to the body, first it comes to the electric aura around the body. A gap appears.

You may be going to have a tumor in the stomach in six months' time. Right now no basis for it exists. No scientist can find anything wrong with your stomach; everything is okay, there is no problem. You can be checked thoroughly and be found all right. But Kirlian photographs the body on a very sensitive plate – he has developed the most sensitive plates. On that plate not only your body is photographed, but also a light aura which you always carry around the body. In that aura, near the stomach, there is a hole. It is not exactly in the physical body, but something is disturbed.

Now he says that he can predict that within six months there will be a tumor. And after six months, when the tumor comes to the body, X-rays will show the same picture he had taken six months before. So Kirlian says that without being ill it can be predicted – if the body aura circulates more, it can be cured before it ever comes to the body, He doesn't know how it can be cured – acupuncture knows, and Patanjali knows.

For Patanjali, disease is some disturbance in the body aura, in the *prana*, the bioenergy, the electricity of your body. That's why it can be cured through om.

Sit alone in a temple sometime, under the dome. You can go to some old temple where nobody goes – a circular dome is just to reflect the sound. Sit under it, chant om loudly, and meditate on it; let the sound reflect back and fall on you like rain and suddenly you will feel after a few minutes that your whole body is becoming peaceful, calm, quiet; the body energy is settling.

The first thing is disease. If you are ill in your *prana* energy, you cannot go far. How can you go far with an illness hanging around you like a cloud? You cannot enter deeper realms. A certain health is needed. The Indian word for health is very meaningful; it is *swasthya*. The very word means to be oneself. The word for health in Sanskrit means to be oneself, to be centered. The English word *health* is also beautiful. It comes from the same word, the same root, from where *holy* and *whole* come. When you are whole you are healthy and when you are whole you are also holy.

It is always good to go to the roots of words because they have arisen out of a long experience of humanity. Words have not come accidentally. When a person feels whole, his body energy is running in a circle. The circle is the most perfect thing in the world. A perfect circle is a symbol of God. Energy is not being wasted, it circulates again and again. It goes on moving like a wheel; it perpetuates itself.

When you are whole you are healthy, and when you are healthy you are also holy because that word *holy* also comes from *whole*. A perfectly healthy person is holy, but there will be problems. If you go to the monasteries you will find all types of sick people there. In fact, only sick people go there. A healthy person – you will question why he is in a monastery. Sick people go there, abnormal people go there. Something is basically wrong with them. That's why they escape from the world and go there.

Patanjali makes it a rule that first you should be healthy because if you are not healthy you cannot go far. Your illness, your discomfort, your broken inner circle of energy will be a stone around your neck. When you meditate you will feel ill at ease. You would like to pray, but you cannot; you would like to rest. You will feel your energy level low, and with low energy you cannot go far. And to reach to God? For Patanjali, God is the farthest point, and much energy is needed. A healthy body, mind, and being is needed. Disease is dis-ease – dis-ease in the body energy. Om will help, and we will also discuss other things. But here Patanjali is talking about how om, the sound itself, helps you to become whole inside.

For Patanjali, and for many others who have searched deeply into human energy, one fact has become very certain – you must know about it – and that is, the more you are ill, the more sensual you become. When you are perfectly healthy you are not sensual. Ordinarily, we think just the contrary – that a healthy man has to be sensual, sexual, this and that; he has to enjoy the world and the body. It is not the case. When you are ill, more sensuality, more sex, grips you. When you are perfectly healthy, sex and sensuality disappear.

Why does it happen so? – because when you are perfectly healthy you are so happy with yourself you don't need the other. When you are ill, you are so unhappy with yourself you need the other. And this is the paradox: when you are ill you need the other, and the other also needs you when she or he is ill. Two people who are ill meeting – the illness is not doubled, it is multiplied.

That's what happens in a marriage: two people who are ill meeting, their illnesses multiply and the whole thing becomes ugly and a hell. People who are ill need others, and they are precisely the people who create trouble when they are relating. A healthy person doesn't need others. But if a healthy person loves, it is not a need, it is a sharing. The whole phenomenon changes. He is not in need of anybody; he has so much that he can share.

A person who is ill needs sex; a healthy person loves. And love is a totally different thing. When two healthy people meet, health is multiplied. They help each other reach for the ultimate. They travel together helping each other to reach for the ultimate. But the need disappears. It is no longer a need, it is no longer a dependence.

Whenever you have an uncomfortable feeling with yourself, don't try to drown it in sex and sensuality. Rather, try to become healthier. *Yogasanas* will help. We will discuss them later on, when Patanjali talks about them. Right now he says, "If you chant om and meditate on it, disease will disappear." He is right. Not only the disease that is present will disappear, but the disease that was to happen in the future will also disappear.

If a man can become a perfect chanting so that the chanter is completely lost – only a pure consciousness, a flame of light, and all around, chanting – the energy falls into a circle, becomes a circle, and you have one of the most euphoric moments in life. When the energy falls into a circle, becomes a harmony, there is no discord, no conflict – you have become one. But ordinarily, disease will be a hindrance. If you are ill, you need treatment.

Patanjali's Yoga system and the Hindu system of medicine, ayurveda, developed simultaneously, together. Ayurveda is totally different to allopathy. Allopathy is suppression of the disease. Allopathy has developed side by side with Christianity; it is a by-product, and because Christianity is suppressive, so is allopathy. If you are ill, allopathy immediately suppresses the illness. The illness will try to come up at some other weak point. It explodes from somewhere else. You suppress it from one place, it explodes from somewhere else. With allopathy you go from one illness to another, and from another to another – it is a never ending process.

Ayurveda has a totally different concept: illness should not be suppressed; it should be released. A catharsis is needed. So ayurvedic medicine is given to the sick person so that the illness comes up and is thrown out, a catharsis. So in the beginning the doses of the ayurvedic medicine may make you more ill, and it takes a long time because it is not a suppression. It cannot be done right now; it is a long process. The illness has to be thrown out and your inner energy has to become a harmony so that the health comes from within. The medicine will throw the illness out, and the healing force will replace it in your own being.

They developed ayurveda and Yoga together. If you are doing *yogaasanas*, and are following Patanjali, never go to an allopathic doctor. If you are not following Patanjali, there is no problem. But if you are following the Yoga system and working many things in your body energy, never have allopathy because they are contrary. Seek an ayurvedic doctor or an homeopath or a naturopath – anything that helps catharsis. If there is a disease, first tackle it; don't move with the disease. With my methods it is very easy to get rid of a disease. Patanjali's method of om, chanting and meditating, is a very mild one… But in those days, that was strong enough because people were simple, they lived with nature. Illness was rare; health was common. Now the case is just the opposite; health is rare, illness is common, and people are very complex, they don't live near nature.

There was a survey carried out in London. One million boys and girls had never seen a cow, they had only seen pictures of one. By and by, we are bracketed into a man-made world: concrete buildings, asphalt roads – all man-made – technology, big machinery, cars. Nature is thrown somewhere into the dark, and nature is a healing force. Man becomes more and more complex. He doesn't listen to his nature; he listens to the demands of civilization, the demands of society. He is completely out of contact with his own inner being.

Patanjali's mild methods won't help much. Hence my dynamic, chaotic methods – because you are almost mad, you need mad methods which can bring out all that is suppressed within you and be thrown out. But health is a must. One who goes for a long journey must make sure that he is healthy. Ill, bedridden, it is difficult to move.

The second obstacle is *languor*. *Languor* means a man who has a very low energy search. He wants to seek and search, but it is a very low energy one – lukewarm. He wants to evaporate, but that's not possible. Such a man always talks about God, *moksha*, Yoga, this and that – but only talks. With a low energy level you can talk; that's all you can do. If you want to do something, you need a high energy effort.

It happened...

Mulla went with his horse and buggy to town. It was a hot summer day, and he was perspiring. Suddenly, the horse stopped on the road, looked back at Mulla and said, "Saints alive, it is too hot!" Mulla could not believe it. He thought he had gone crazy because of the heat. How could the horse talk?

So he looked around to see if anybody else had heard, but there was nobody except his dog, who was sitting in the buggy. Not finding anyone, but just to get rid of the idea, he said to the dog, "Did you hear what he said?"

The dog replied, "Oh, he is just like everyone else – always talking about the weather and doing nothing."

This is the man of languor – always talking about God, and doing nothing. He always talks of great things, but this talk is just to hide a wound. He talks so that he can forget that he is not doing anything about it. He escapes through a cloud of talk. Talking about it again and again, he thinks he is doing something, but talk is not a doing. You can go on talking about the weather, you can go on talking about God – if you don't do anything, you are simply wasting your energy.

This type of person can become a minister, a priest, a pundit. These are low energy people. They become very proficient at talking – so proficient that they can deceive you because they always talk about beautiful and great things. Others listen to them and get deceived. Philosophers – they are all people of languor. Patanjali is not a philosopher. He himself is a scientist, and he wants others to be scientists. Much effort is needed.

Through the chanting of om and meditating on it, your low energy level will become high. How does it happen? Why is your energy always at a low level, making you feel exhausted, tired? Even in the morning when you get up you are tired. What is happening to you? – somewhere in your system there are leakages; you leak energy. You are not aware of it, but you are like a bucket with holes. Every day you fill the bucket, but notice that it is always emptying. This leakage has to be stopped.

How does energy leak through the body? These are deep problems for bioenergetics. The body always leaks energy through the fingers, feet, and eyes. The energy cannot leak through the head because it is round. Anything round in shape helps the body to preserve energy. That's why yoga postures – *siddhasana, padmasana* – make the whole body round.

A person who is sitting in a *siddhasana* puts both his hands together because the body energy leaks through the fingers. When both hands are put together one on top of each other, the energy moves from one hand into the other. It becomes a circle. The feet and legs are also put on top of each other so that the energy moves in your own body and doesn't leak.

The eyes are closed because the eyes release almost eighty percent of your bioenergy. That's why, if you are on a journey and go on looking out of the train or the car, you will feel so tired. If you travel with closed eyes, you will not feel so tired. You go on looking at unnecessary things, even reading advertisements on the walls. You use your eyes too much, and when the eyes are tired the whole body is tired. The eyes give the indication that now it is enough A yogi tries to remain as much as possible with closed eyes, and with his hands and legs crossing each other, so the energy moves into each. He sits with his spine straight. If your spine is straight while you are sitting you will preserve more energy than any other way – because when the spine is straight, the gravitation of the earth cannot force much energy out of you, as it touches only one point of the spine. When you are sitting and leaning, your body slanting, you think you are resting, but Patanjali says that you are leaking energy because more of your body is under the influence of gravitation. This won't help.

With a straight spine, closed hands and legs, and closed eyes, you have become a circle; that circle is represented by *shivalinga*. You must have seen the *shivalinga* – the phallic symbol, as it is known in the West. In fact, it is the inner bioenergy circle, just egg shaped. When your body energy flows rightly, it becomes like an egg; the shape is an egg, exactly like an egg, and that is symbolized in the *shivalinga*. You become a Shiva. When the energy is flowing into yourself again and again, and not moving out, languor disappears. It will not disappear by talking; it will not disappear by reading scriptures; it will not disappear by philosophizing. It will disappear only when your energy is not leaking.

Try to preserve it. The more you preserve, the better. But in the West something just the opposite is being taught: that it is good to release energy through sex, and this and that – to release energy. It is good if you are not using it in any other way, otherwise you will go mad. Whenever there is too much energy, it is better to release it through sex. Sex is the simplest method to release it.

But it can be used. It can be made creative. It can give you a rebirth, a resurrection. You can know millions of euphoric stages through it; you can rise higher and higher through it. It is the ladder to reach godliness. If you go on releasing it every day, you will never build up enough energy to take even the first step toward the divine. Preserve!

Patanjali is against sex, and that is the difference between Patanjali and Tantra. Tantra uses sex as a method; Patanjali wants you to bypass it. And there are people, almost fifty percent, to whom Tantra will suit; and fifty percent to whom Yoga will suit. One has to find what will suit you. Both can be used, and through both, people reach. Neither is wrong or right, it depends on you. One will be right for you and one will be wrong for you, but remember, for *you*! It is not an absolute categorical statement.

Something may be right for you and wrong for somebody else. Both the systems were born together, Tantra and Yoga – twin systems, exactly at the same time – this is the synchronicity. As man and woman need each other, Tantra and Yoga need each other; they become a complete thing. If there is only Yoga, only fifty percent can reach; the other fifty percent will be in trouble. If there is only Tantra, fifty percent can reach; the other fifty percent will be in trouble. This has happened.

Sometimes, not knowing where you are moving to – or what you are doing, and not knowing who you are and what will suit you – you go on without a master. You may be a woman and dressed like a man, and think of yourself as a man; you will be in trouble. You may be a man and dressed like a woman, and think of yourself as a woman; you will be in trouble.

Trouble arises when you don't understand who you are. A master is needed to give you a clear-cut direction that "This is for you." So remember, whenever I say that something is for you, don't go on spreading it to others because it has been specifically told to you. People are curious. If you tell them, they will try. It may not be for them. It may even be harmful. Remember, if it is not helpful, it is going to be harmful. There is no in between. Something is either helpful for you or harmful.

Languor is one of the greatest obstacles, but it disappears through the chanting of om. The om creates the *shivalinga* within you, the egg shaped energy circle. When you become perceptive you can even see it. If you chant om for a few months with your eyes closed and meditate, you can see within yourself;

your body has disappeared. There will be just a bioenergy, an electric phenomenon, and the shape will be that of the *shivalinga*.

The moment this happens to you, languor has disappeared. Now you are a high energy, now you can move mountains. You feel that talking is not enough, something has to be done. The energy level is so high that something can be done now. People come to me and ask, "What to do," but I look at them and see that they are leaking energy; they cannot do anything. The first thing is to drop this leakage. Only ask "What can be done" when you have energy.

Doubt: Sanskrit has many words it. English has only one word for it. So try to understand, and I will explain it to you. There is a doubt against trust; in Sanskrit it is called *shanka* – doubt against trust, one pair. There is a doubt called *sanshaya* – Patanjali is talking about *sanshaya* now – doubt against certainty, against decisiveness. A man of uncertainty who is not decisive is in *sanshaya*, in doubt. This is not against trust, because *trust* is to trust in somebody. This is against self-confidence; you don't trust in yourself. That's a different thing.

So whatever you do, you are not certain whether you want to do it or not, whether it will be good to go into it or not – an indecisiveness. With an indecisive mind you cannot enter on the path – not on the path of Patanjali. You have to be decisive. You have to make a decision. It is difficult because a part of you always goes on saying no. How to make the decision? – think about it as much as you can; give it as much time as you can. Think of all the possibilities, all the alternatives, and decide. Once you decide, drop all doubting.

Before that, use it and do whatever you can do with the doubt. Think of all the possibilities and choose. Of course, it is not going to be a total decision; in the beginning it is not possible. It will be a majority decision – the majority of your mind will say yes. Once you decide, never doubt. Doubt will raise its head. You simply say, "I have decided – finished! It is not a total

THE HEART OF YOGA

decision, all the doubts are not discarded, but whatever could be done, I have done. I have thought it out as completely as possible and I have chosen."

Once you choose, never give doubt any cooperation again – doubt exists in you with your cooperation. You go on giving energy to it, and you start thinking about it again and again. An indecisiveness is created. Indecisiveness is a very bad state of affairs – you are in very bad shape. If you cannot decide anything, how can you do it? How can you act?

How will om, the sound and the meditation, help? – it helps because once you become silent, peaceful, a decision becomes easier. You are no longer a crowd, and not in chaos with many voices talking together and not knowing which voice is yours. With the chanting of om, the meditating on it, the voices become silent. Many voices – now you can see they are not yours – your mother, your father, your brothers, your teachers are speaking; they are not yours. You can discard them easily because they don't need any attention.

When you become silent under the chanting of om you are sheltered, calm, quiet, collected. In that collectedness you can see which is the real voice coming from you, which is the authentic one. It is as if you are standing in a marketplace and many people are talking and many things are going on, and you cannot decide what is happening. On a stock market, people are shouting – they know their language but you cannot understand what is happening, whether they have gone mad or not. You move to a Himalayan retreat. You sit in a cave, and simply chant. You simply calm yourself down, all nervousness disappears; you become one, collected. In that moment, decisiveness is possible – then decide, and don't look back. Forget – it is decided. Now there is no going back. Now go ahead.

Sometimes the doubt will follow you and bark at you like a dog. But if you don't listen and don't pay attention, by and by it stops. Give it a chance, think all that is possible and, once decided, drop it. *Omkar* will help you to come to a decisiveness. Here, *doubt* means indecisiveness.

Carelessness: the Sanskrit word for it is *pramad. Pramad* means as if one is walking in sleep. Carelessness is part of it; an exact translation would be, "Don't be a zombie; don't walk in hypnosis." But you live as if in an hypnotic state, not knowing it at all. The whole of society is trying to hypnotize you for certain things, and that creates *pramad,* that creates a sleepiness in you. What is happening? – you are not aware, otherwise you would be simply surprised by what is happening. It is so familiar, that's why you don't become aware of it. You are being pulled by many manipulators, and their method of manipulation is by creating an hypnotic state in you.

For example, they go on advertising a certain thing on the radio, on the TV, in the cinema, and in every newspaper and magazine – "Lux toilet soap." You think you are not affected, but every day you hear, "Lux toilet soap, Lux toilet soap, Lux toilet soap." It is a chant. At night, on the streets, neon lights say "Lux toilet soap." And now they have found out that it is more impressive if you make the lights flicker. If it goes on and off, it is even more impressive because you have to read it again: "Lux toilet soap." The light goes off, comes on again, and you have to read it again: "Lux toilet soap."

You are chanting om; it is going deeper into your subconscious. You think you are not bothered, you think you are not befooled by these people – all these beautiful naked women standing near Lux toilet soap and saying, "Why am I beautiful? Why is my face so beautiful? – because of Lux toilet soap." You know that you are not beautiful, but you are affected. Suddenly, one day you go to a shop in the market and ask for soap. The shopkeeper asks, "Which soap?" Suddenly it bubbles up: "Lux toilet soap."

You are being hypnotized by the businessmen, political leaders, educationists, priests because everybody has an investment in you being hypnotized. Then you can be used. The politicians go on saying, "This is your mother country, and if your mother country is in difficulty, go to war and become a martyr."

What nonsense! The whole earth is your mother. Is the earth divided into India, Pakistan, Germany, England – or is it one? But the politicians are continuously hammering on your mind that only this part of the earth is your mother; you have to save it. Even if you lose your life, it is very good. And they go on: devotion to the country, nationalism, patriotism – all nonsense terms, but if you are hammered continuously you become hypnotized. You can sacrifice yourself.

You are sacrificing your life in an hypnotic state because of slogans. Through hypnosis a flag, an ordinary piece of cloth, becomes so important. "This is our national flag." Millions die for it. If there are beings on other planets and if sometimes they look at the earth, they will think, "These people are simply mad." For a cloth – a piece of cloth – because you have insulted "our flag," and this cannot be tolerated...

Religions go on preaching that you are a Christian, a Hindu, a Mohammedan, this and that, and they make you feel that you are a Christian on a crusade: "Kill others who are not Christians. This is your duty!" They teach you such absurd things, but you still believe it because they go on saying it. Adolf Hitler says in his autobiography, *Mein Kampf*, that if you repeat a lie continuously it becomes a truth. And he knows; nobody knows as well as he does because he repeated lies himself and created the phenomenon.

Pramad means a state of hypnosis, manipulated, moving sleepily. And because you are not yourself, carelessness is bound to happen and you do everything without any care. You move and stumble on. In relationship with things, with people, you are continuously stumbling about; you are not going anywhere, you are just like a drunkard. But everybody else is just like you, so you don't have the opportunity to feel that you are a drunkard.

Be careful. How will om help you to be careful? – the

hypnosis will drop. In fact, if you simply chant om without meditating, it will also become a hypnosis; that's the difference between the ordinary chanting of a mantra and Patanjali's way. Chant it and remain aware. If you chant om and remain aware, the om and its chanting will become a dehypnotizing force. It will destroy all the hypnosis that exists around you, that has been created in you by the society and the manipulators, the politicians. It will be a dehypnotization.

In America, somebody asked Vivekananda, "What is the difference between ordinary hypnosis and your chanting of om?" He said, "The chanting of om is a dehypnosis; it is moving in reverse gear." The process seems to be the same, but the gear is in reverse. How does it reverse? – if you are meditating, by and by you become so silent and so aware, so careful, that nobody can hypnotize you. Now you are beyond the reach of priests and politicians – the poisoners. Now, for the first time, you are an individual, and you become careful. You move with care, being careful with each step because there are millions of pitfalls all around you.

Laziness: alasya. So much laziness has accumulated in you. It comes for certain reasons – because you don't see the point of doing anything, and even if you do, nothing is achieved. If you don't do anything, nothing is lost. A laziness settles in the heart. Laziness simply means that you have lost the zest for life.

Children are not lazy, they are bubbling with energy. You have to force them to go to sleep; you have to force them to be silent; you have to force them to sit for a few minutes in order to relax. They are not tense; this is your idea. They are full of energy – such tiny beings with so much energy! From where does this energy come? – they are still unfrustrated. They don't know that in this life, whatever you do, nothing is achieved. They are unaware – blissfully unaware; that's why they have so much energy.

You have been doing many things, and nothing is achieved. Laziness settles. It is like dust settling in you – of all the failures, frustrations, of every dream gone sour. It settles. You become lazy. In the morning, you think, "Why do I need to get up again? What for?" There is no answer. You have to get up because somehow bread has to be earned. There is a wife, and children; you are caught in the trap. You travel to the office somehow; you come back somehow. There is no zest in your life; you drag. You are not happy doing anything.

How will the chanting of om and meditating on it help? – it helps, certainly helps because when you chant om and watch and meditate for the first time, this first effort in your life seems to bring a fulfillment. You feel so happy and blissful chanting it, that this first effort has succeeded. Now a new zest arises. The dust is being thrown off. A new courage, a new confidence is attained. Now you think that you can also do something, and can also achieve something. Everything is not a failure. Maybe the outward journey is a failure, but the inward journey is not. Even the first step brings so many flowers. Now hope arises, and confidence settles again. You are again a child – of the inner world. A new birth. You can laugh, run, play again. You are born again.

This is what Hindus call the twice-born. This is the next birth, a second birth. The first birth was in the outside world. It has proved a failure; that's why you feel so lethargic. By the time one is forty, one starts thinking of death – how to die, how to be finished. If people don't commit suicide, it is not that they are happy. It is only because even in death they simply don't see any hope. Even death seems to be hopeless. It is not because they love life that they are not committing suicide, no. They are so frustrated because they know that even death is not going to give anything. So why commit suicide unnecessarily? Why take the trouble? So they go on as things are.

Sensuality: Why do you feel sensual, sexual? – you feel sexual because you accumulate energy, unused energy, and you don't know what to do with it. So, naturally, it accumulates at the first center, sex. You don't know any other centers, and you don't know how it can flow upward. It's like when you have an airplane, but you don't know what it is. So you look into it, and think, "It has wheels, so it must be a sort of vehicle." So you yoke some horses to it and use it as a bullock cart. It can be used. Someday, just by accident, you discover that the bullocks aren't needed. It has a certain type of engine in it, so you use it as a motorcar. Then you look deeper and deeper into it, and wonder: "What are these wings for?" One day you use it as it should be used – as an airplane.

When you move inside yourself, you discover many things. But if you don't move, there is only sexuality. You gather energy – what to do with it? You don't know anything; you don't know that you can fly upward. You become a bullock cart; sex is behaving like a bullock cart. You gather energy by eating food, drinking water. When energy is created, and available, if you don't use it, you will go mad. The energy travels round and round within you. It makes you crazy. You have to do something. If you don't do something, you will go crazy; you will explode. Sex is the easiest safety valve – the energy moves back into nature.

This is foolish because the energy comes from nature. You eat food; it is eating nature. You drink water; it is drinking nature. You sunbathe; it is eating the sun. You are continuously eating nature, and throw it back out to nature. The whole thing seems to be baseless, useless, with no meaning. What's the use of it all? You become lethargic.

Energy must go higher. You must become a transformer; through you nature must become supernature, only then is there meaning, significance. Through you matter must become the mind; the mind must become the supermind. Through you nature must reach to supernature; the lowest must become the highest. Only then there is a significance, a felt significance. Your life then has a deep, deep significance. You are not worthless, you are not like dirt; you are a god! When you have moved nature through you, to supernature, you have become a god – Patanjali's god. You become a master of masters.

But ordinarily, sensuality means that energy has built up and you have to throw it out. You don't know what to do with it. First you gather it together. You go on seeking food, and using a lot of effort to earn your bread. You absorb the bread and create energy. And sexual energy is the most refined in your body – the most refined. You throw it out, and enter again into the circle. It is a vicious circle. When you throw it out, the body needs energy again. You eat, collect, throw it. So how can you feel that you have some meaning? You seem to be in a rut leading nowhere. How will om help? How will meditating on it help? – once you start meditating on om, other centers start functioning.

When the energy flows, it becomes a circle inside you. The sex center is not the only center which is functioning. Your whole body becomes a circle. From the sex center it rises to the second, to the third, fourth, fifth, sixth, seventh center; then again sixth, fifth, fourth, third, second, first. It becomes an inner circle and it passes other centers.

As energy is accumulated, it rises higher. The level rises higher, just like a dam; the water keeps coming in from the river, and the dam is not allowing it to flow out. The water rises high and other centers, other chakras in your body start opening – because when the energy flows they become dynamic forces, dynamos. They start functioning. It is as if a waterfall and a dynamo start functioning. When the waterfall is dry, the dynamo cannot start. When the energy flows upward, your highest chakras start working, functioning. This is how om helps. It makes you calm, collected, one. Energy rises high; sensuality disappears. Sex becomes meaningless, childish; not yet gone, but it becomes childish. You don't feel sensual; you don't feel any urge for it.

It is still there, and if you are not careful, it will have you in its grip again. You can fall, because this is not the ultimate happening. You are not yet crystallized, but a glimpse has happened – that the energy can give you inner ecstatic states. Sex is the lowest ecstasy. Higher ecstasies are possible. When the higher becomes possible, the lower automatically disappears. You need not renounce it. If you renounce it, your energy will not move higher; if the energy is moving higher, there is no need to renounce it. It simply becomes useless, and drops by itself. It becomes nonfunctioning.

Delusion: as you are, psychoanalysts say that if you stop dreaming you will go mad. Dreams are needed because in your state of mind delusions are needed. Delusions, deceptions, illusions – dreams are needed because you are sleepy, and dreams are a necessity in sleep.

In America they have been experimenting. If you are stopped from dreaming for seven days, you immediately start experiencing a delusional trip; with your eyes open you start seeing things which are not there. You start talking to people who are not there, and you start having visions. You are mad. Just seven days of no dreaming and you become delusionary; hallucinations start happening. Your dreams are a catharsis, an inbuilt catharsis, so every night you delude yourself. By morning you are a little sober, but again by the evening you have gathered so much energy. At night you have to dream and throw it out.

This happens to drivers, and many accidents happen because of it. Accidents happen at night, around four o'clock in the morning because the driver has been driving the whole night through. He has not been dreaming, but the dream energy accumulates. He is driving with his eyes open and he starts having illusions. He says to himself, "The road is straight. There is nobody on the road, no truck is coming." With his eyes open he drives into a truck. Or he sees a truck coming – when there isn't one. Just to avoid it, he crashes against a tree.

A lot of research has been done on why so many accidents happen about four in the morning. In fact, about four in the morning you dream too much. At four, five, six o'clock, you dream too much! That is dream time. You have slept well; now there is no need for sleep, you can dream. In the morning you dream, and at that time if you don't dream, or you are not allowed to, you will create delusions. You will dream with open eyes.

Delusion means dreaming with open eyes, but everybody is dreaming that way. For example: you see a woman and think she is absolutely beautiful. That may or maybe not be the case. You may be having an illusion and projecting it on her. You may be sexually starved, and because of that energy, you delude yourself. After two or three days, the woman looks ordinary, and you think you have been deceived. Nobody is deceiving you, only you yourself. But you have deluded others. Lovers delude each other, they dream with open eyes and become frustrated. Nobody is at fault, just your state.

Patanjali says, "Delusion will disappear if you chant om with mindfulness." How will it happen? Delusion means a dreaming state: when you are lost, you are no longer there; there is just the dream. If you meditate on om, and when you have created the sound of om and you are a witness, you are there. Your presence will not allow any dreams to happen.

Whenever you are, there is no dream. Whenever there is a dream, you are not. You cannot be both together. If you are there the dream will disappear – or you will have to disappear. Both cannot be together. Dream and awareness never meet. That's why delusion disappears by witnessing the sound of om.

Impotency: impotency is felt continuously. You feel yourself helpless; that is impotency. You feel you cannot do anything, that you are worthless, of no use. You may pretend that you are somebody, but your pretension shows that deep down you feel nobodyness. You may pretend that you are very powerful, but you are hiding in that pretension.

Mulla Nasruddin entered a bar with a sheet of paper in his hand and declared, "Here are the names of the people I can lick" – a hundred names.

One man stood up. He was a tiny man; Mulla could have

licked him. But he had two pistols in his belt. He came near with a pistol in his hand and said, "Is my name also there?"

Mulla looked at him and said, "Yes."

The man said, "You cannot lick me."

Mulla replied, "Are you sure?"

The man said, "Absolutely. Look!" And he showed him the pistol.

Mulla said, "Okay. I will take your name off the list."

You can pretend you are very powerful, but whenever you are in an encounter you start feeling helpless and powerless. Man is impotent because only the whole can be potent, not man. The part cannot be potent. Only God is potent; man is impotent.

When you chant *omkar*, om, for the first time you feel that you are no longer an island. You become one part of the whole universal sound. For the first time you feel yourself potent, but now this potency need not be violent, need not be aggressive. In fact, a powerful man is never aggressive. Only impotent people become aggressive to prove to themselves: "We are powerful."

...and instability are the obstacles that distract the mind. You start one thing and stop. You are on and off; you start again and then you're off. Nothing is possible with this instability. One has to persevere, and go on continuously digging the hole at the same spot. If you stop your effort, your mind is such that after a few days you will have to start from *ABC* again; it rewinds itself, it unwinds itself. You do something for a few days, and then you leave it. You will be thrown back to the first day of your doing, back again to *ABC*. You can do so much without achieving anything. Om will give you a taste.

Why do you start and stop? People come to me and tell me that they have meditated for a year, and stopped. When I ask them, "How were you feeling?" They reply, "We were feeling very, very good" – so why did you stop? Nobody stops when they are feeling very, very good. They continue, "We were very happy and we stopped." It is impossible! If you were happy, how can you stop? Then they say, "Not exactly happy…"

They are in trouble because they even pretend that they are happy. If you are happy in a certain thing you continue with it. You stop only when it is boring, an unhappiness. About om, Patanjali says, "You will feel the first taste of dropping into the universal. That taste will become your happiness and instability will go." That's why he says, "Through chanting om and witnessing it, all obstacles drop."

> Anguish, despair, tremors and irregular breathing are
> the symptoms of a distracted mind.

These are the symptoms. *Anguish*: always anxiety ridden, always split, with an anxious mind, always sad – in *despair*. There are subtle *tremors* in the body energy because when the body energy is not running in a circle you have subtle tremors, a trembling, fear …*and irregular breathing…* Your breathing cannot be a rhythm, it cannot be a song, it cannot be a harmony – an *irregular breathing…*

These …*are the symptoms of a distracted mind.* And against these are the symptoms of a mind that is centered. Chanting om will make you centered. Your breathing will become rhythmic. Your body tremors will disappear; you will not be nervous. Sadness will be replaced by a feeling of happiness, joy, with a subtle blissfulness on your face – for no reason at all. You are simply happy; just being here you are happy, just breathing you are happy. You don't demand much, and instead of anguish there will be bliss.

> To remove these, meditate on one principle.

These symptoms of a distracted mind can be removed by meditating on one principle. That one principle is *pranava*, om, the universal sound.

Enough for today.

8

Death Is an Alchemy

The first question:

Osho,
The path seems to be toward peace and awareness.
Why then is everyone and everything around you in
such a chaos?

I am a chaos, and only out of a chaos is a cosmos born; there is
no other way. You are like very old, ancient buildings; you cannot
be renovated. You have been here for millions of lives. First you
have to be demolished completely, and only then recreated.

Renovation is possible, but that won't help for long. It will just
be surface decoration. Deep in your foundations you will remain
with the old and the whole structure will always remain shaky and
can fall any day. New foundations are needed – everything has to
be new. You have to be completely reborn, otherwise it will be a
modification. You can be painted from the outside, but there is
no way to paint the inner. The inner will remain the same – the
same old rotten thing.

A discontinuity is needed. You should not be allowed to continue. The old simply dies and the new comes out of it, out of
the death. There is a gap between the old and the new; otherwise

the old can continue. All modifications are really to save the old, and I am not a modifier. The chaos will continue if you resist it, and it will take a long time.

If you allow it to happen, it can happen in a single moment. If you allow it to happen, the old disappears and a new being emerges. That new being will be divine because it will not come out of the past, it will not come out of time. It will be timeless – beyond time. It will not come out of *you*, you will not be a father and mother to it. It will come suddenly out of the blue. That's why Buddha insists that it always comes out of nothing.

You are something; that is the misery. What are you in fact? – just the past. You go on accumulating the past; that's why you have become like ruins – very ancient ones. Just see the point and don't try to continue with the old. Drop it! Hence, around me there is always going to be chaos because I am continuously demolishing. I am destructive because that is the only way to be creative. I am like death because only then can you be born through me. It is right, there is chaos. There always will be – it will continue because new people will be coming. You will never find a settled establishment around me. New people will be coming and I will be demolishing them.

It can stop for you individually; the chaos will disappear if you allow me to destroy you completely. You will become a cosmos, a hidden harmony, a deep order. The chaos will disappear for you, but around me it will continue because new people will be coming. This has to be so, this has always been so.

It is not the first time that you have asked me this. Buddha was asked the same, and Lao Tzu also; the same will be asked again and again because whenever there is a master... That means he uses death as a method for resurrection. You must die; only then you can be reborn.

Chaos is beautiful because it is the womb; your so-called order is ugly because it protects only the dead. Death is beautiful, dead is not – remember the difference. I repeat, "Death is beautiful because it is an alive force. Dead is not beautiful because it is that place from where life has already moved. It is just a ruin." Don't be a dead one; don't carry the past. Drop it, and pass through death. You are afraid of death, but you are not afraid of the dead.

Jesus called out to two fishermen to follow him, and the moment they were leaving the town a man came running up to them and said, "Where are you going? Your father has died. Come back."

They asked Jesus, "Allow us a few days so that we can go and do whatever is needed. Our father is dead and the last rituals have to be carried out."

Jesus replied, "Let the dead bury their dead – don't bother, follow me."

What is Jesus saying? – he is saying that the whole town is dead, they'll take care of it: "Let the dead bury their dead. Follow me."

If you live in the past you are a dead thing, you are not an alive force. There is only one way to become alive, and that is to die to the past, die to the dead. This is not going to happen once and forever. Once you know the secret that each moment you have to die to the past so no dust gathers on you, death then becomes a constant reorientation, a constant rebirth.

Always remember: die to the past. Whatever has passed has passed. It is no more; it is nowhere. It only clings in the memory, it is only in your mind. The mind is the repository of all that is dead. That's why only the mind is the block for life to flow. The dead bodies accumulate around the flow, and they become the block.

All that I am doing here is helping you to learn how to die because that's the first aspect of how to be reborn. Death is beautiful because life comes out of it fresh like dewdrops. So chaos is being used, and you will feel it around me. And that will always be so because somewhere or other I am demolishing somebody – in thousands of ways, known or unknown to you, I am demolishing you. I am shaking you out of your death, shaking you out of your past, trying to make you more aware and more alive.

In the ancient Hindu scriptures it is said that a master is a death. They knew that a master has to be a death because out of that death comes revolution, mutation, transformation, transcendence. Death is an alchemy – it is the most subtle alchemy, and nature uses it. When somebody becomes very old, ancient, nature kills him.

You are afraid because you cling to the past. Otherwise you would be happy, and would welcome it – you would feel grateful to nature because nature always kills the old, the past, the dead, and your life moves into a new body. An old man becomes a new baby, completely clean of the past. That's why nature helps you not to remember the past. Nature uses ways to allow you not to remember the past; otherwise you will be old the very moment you are born. The old man dies and is born as a new baby, but if he can remember the past he will be already old; the whole purpose will be lost.

Nature closes the past for you, so every birth seems to be a new birth. But you start accumulating again. When it is too much, nature will kill you again. One becomes capable of knowing past lives only when one is dead to the past. Then nature opens the door. Nature knows and there is no need for nature to hide from you. You have attained the constant newness, freshness of life. Now you know how to die, nature need not kill you.

Once you know that you are not the past, that you are not the future, but you are the very "presentness" of things, the whole of nature opens its doors and mysteries. Your whole past – millions of lives lived in many, many ways – is revealed. Now it can be revealed because you will not be burdened by it. Now the past can't burden you. If you come to know the alchemy of how to become continuously new, this will be your last life because there is no need to kill you and help you to be reborn. There is no need. You are doing it yourself every moment.

That's the meaning when a buddha disappears and never comes back, and why an enlightened person is never born again. That is the secret: now he knows death, and continuously uses it. Every moment whatever is past, is past and dead, and he is freed of it. Every moment he dies to the past and is born anew. It becomes a constant flow, a riverlike flow of gaining fresh life every moment. There is no need for nature to gather seventy years of nonsense, rubbish, rot, and to kill this ruin of a man and help him to be born again, and to put him in the same circle – because he will gather it all again.

This is a vicious circle. Hindus have called it the *sansar*. *Sansar* means the wheel; the wheel goes on moving again and again on the same route. An enlightened person is one who has dropped out of the wheel. He says, "No more of it! Nature need not kill me – now I kill myself every moment."

If you are fresh, nature need not use death for you – and there is no need for birth, because you are continuously using birth. Every moment you die to the past and are born to the present. That's why you feel a subtle freshness around a buddha, as if he has just taken a bath. You come close to him and feel a fragrance – a fragrance of freshness. You can never meet the same buddha again. Every moment he is new.

Hindus are very wise because in thousands of years of encountering buddhas, *jinas* – conquerors of life, enlightened, awakened people – they have realized many truths. One of the truths you will see all around: no Buddha, no Mahavira is depicted as old. Krishna, Rama, Buddha, Mahavira – no statue, no picture exists… Nobody is depicted as old.

Not that they never became old; they became old. Buddha became old – he was eighty. He was as old as anybody would be on becoming eighty, but he is not depicted as old. The reason is inner. Whenever you came near to him you would find him young and fresh. So the oldness was just in the body, not in him. I have to demolish you because your body may be young, but your inner being is very, very old and ancient – a ruin, just like the Iranian ruins of Persepolis and others.

Inside, you have a ruin of a being. It has to be demolished – I have to be a furnace, a fire, a death to you. That's the only way I can help and bring a cosmos within you, an order. I am not working to enforce any order upon you because that won't help. Any order enforced from without will be just a prop for the old ancient ruin, and it will not help.

I believe in an inner order. That happens with your own awareness and rebirth. That comes from within and spreads outward. It opens just like a flower, the petals move outward from the center to the periphery. Only that order which opens within you and spreads all around is real and beautiful. If order is enforced from without, if a discipline is given to you – "Do this and don't do that" – and you are forced to be a prisoner, that won't help because it won't change you.

Nothing can change from the outside. There is only one revolution; that which comes from within. But before that revolution happens you must be utterly destroyed. Only on your grave will the new be born. That's why there is chaos around me – because I am a chaos, and I am using chaos as a method.

The second question:

Osho,
In doing *sadhana*, meditation, on om, is it better to repeat it like a mantra or to try to hear it as an inner sound?

The mantra om has to be done in three stages. First, you should repeat it very loudly. That means it should come from the body – first from the body because it is the main door. Let the body be saturated with it.

So repeat it loudly. Go to a temple or to your room or some-where where you can repeat it as loudly as you like. Use the whole body to repeat it, as if thousands of people are listening to you and you are not using a microphone; you have to be very loud so that the whole body trembles, and shakes with it. For almost three months, you should not bother about anything else. The first stage is very important because it gives the foundation. So loudly, as if every cell of your body is crying it, chanting it.

After three months, when you feel your body is completely saturated, and it has entered deep down into the body cells – and when you say it loudly, it is not only coming from the mouth, the whole body is repeating it... From the head to the toe, it comes! If you repeat it continuously for at least one hour a day for three months, within three months you will feel that it is not the mouth alone, it is the whole body. It happens – it has happened many times.

If you do it honestly, authentically, not deceiving yourself, and if it is not lukewarm but a hundred-degree phenomenon, then even others can listen. They can put their ears to your feet, and when you say it loudly they will hear it coming from your bones because the whole body can absorb and create sound. There are no problems. Your mouth is just a part of the body, a specialized part, that's all. If you try, your whole body can repeat it.

It happened...

A Hindu sannyasin, Swami Ram, chanted "Ram" loudly for many years. Once he was staying in a Himalayan village with a friend. The friend was a very well-known Sikh writer, Sardar Purnasingh. In the middle of the night Purnasingh suddenly heard chanting: "Ram, Ram, Ram." There was nobody else – only Ram, Swami Ram, and himself. They were both asleep in their beds, and the village was far away – almost two, three miles away. There was nobody else.

So Purnasingh got up, and walked around the cottage; there was nobody else there. As he went farther away from Ram, the sound became less and less. When he came back, the sound became louder. The moment he came nearer to Ram, who was fast asleep, the sound became even louder. He put his ear to Ram's body; the whole of his body was vibrating with the sound of "Ram."

It happens – your whole body can become saturated. This is the first step – three, six months – but you must feel saturated. The saturation feels like when you are hungry and you eat some food – the feeling when the stomach is satisfied. The body must be satisfied first, and if you continue, it may happen in three or six months. Three months is the average time; for a few people it happens even before, and for a few it takes a little more time.

If it saturates the whole body, sex will completely disappear. The whole body is so soothed, it becomes so calm with the vibrating sound that there is no need to throw the energy out; there is no need to release it, and you will feel very, very powerful. But don't use this power – because you can use it, but all use will be misuse. This is just a first step. The energy has to be gathered so that you can take the second step. If you choose to use it, you can because the power will be so much that you can do many things – you can simply say something and it will come true. But at this stage it has been prohibited; you should not be active, and you should not say anything. You should not say something to someone in anger, for instance: "Go and die," because it can happen. Your sound becomes so powerful when it is saturated with your whole body energy that it is said that at this stage negative things should not be said. Even unknowingly, negative things should not be said.

You may be surprised, but it is good that I tell you: "We were building a roof at the back of this house; it fell down. It fell down because of some of you." You are making a tremendous effort in meditation, and there are at least twenty people who were thinking that it would fall down. They helped; they helped it to fall down. At least twenty people were continuously thinking about it. When they looked at it, they thought it would fall because of its shape and to their minds it was unlikely that it was going to remain as it was.

It fell! And when it fell, they thought, "Of course we were right." This is the vicious circle. You are the cause! – and you think you were right. And you are all putting so much effort into your meditation that whatever you think can happen. Never think a negative thought when you are meditating. It is possible – because you gain some power. But I am not concerned that the roof fell. But because of its falling many of you have lost a certain quantity of power; that is more of a concern to me because nothing happens without your power being used in it.

There were those who were saying that the roof would fall down, and it fell. They could see themselves; for a few days they remained very impotent, sad, depressed. They lost their power. They may have been thinking that they were sad because the roof had fallen down – no! They were sad because they had lost a certain quantity of power, and life is an energy phenomenon.

When you don't meditate, there is not much of a problem. You can say whatever you like because you are impotent. But when you meditate, you should be watchful of every single word that you say because every single word can create something around you.

The first step is to saturate the whole body, so that it becomes a chanting force. When you feel satisfied, take the second step. Never use this power, because it has to be accumulated and to be used for the second step. The second step is to close your mouth and repeat and chant the word *om* mentally. First bodily, second mentally. Now the body should not be used at all. The throat, tongue, lips – everything closed. The whole body locked, and the chanting only happening in the mind, but as loudly as possible –

the same loudness as you were using with the body. Now let the mind be saturated with it. Again for three months, let the mind be saturated with it.

It takes the same time for the mind as it does for the body. If you can attain the saturation within one month with the body, you will also attain in one month with the mind. If you attain in seven months with the body, you will attain in seven months with the mind because body and mind are not exactly two; they are rather body-mind, a psychosomatic phenomenon. One part is the body, the other part is the mind; body is visible mind, mind is invisible body.

Let the other part, the subtle part of your personality, be saturated; repeat loudly inside. When the mind is filled, even more power is released within you. With the first, sex will disappear; with the second, love will disappear – the love that you know, not the love that a buddha knows, but your love will disappear. Sex is the bodily part of love and love is the mental part of sex. When love disappears, there is even more danger. You can be fatal to others. If you say something, it will happen immediately. That's why total silence is proposed for the second stage. So when you are in the second stage, be completely silent.

There will be a tendency to use the power because you will be very curious about it, childish, and you will have so much energy that you would like to see what could happen if you used it. But don't use it and don't be juvenile because the third step still has to be taken and energy is needed for that. That's why sex disappeared – because the energy has to be accumulated; love disappeared – because subtle energy has to be accumulated.

The third step is when the mind feels saturated – and you will know when this happens; there is no need to ask how one will feel it. It is just like when you are eating you feel, "Now, that's enough." The mind will feel when it is enough. Then you start the third step. The third step is that neither the body nor the mind has to be used. As you lock the body, now you lock the mind.

It is easy. When you have been doing the chanting for three, four months, it is very easy; you simply lock the body, lock the mind. Just listen – you will hear a sound coming to you from your own heart of hearts. The om will be there as if somebody else is chanting; you are just the listener. This is the third step, and this third step will change your total being. All the barriers will drop and all the obstacles will disappear. If you put your total energy in it, on average, it can take almost nine months.

You say: "In doing *sadhana*, meditation, on om, is it better to repeat it like a mantra or to try to hear it as an inner sound?" Right now you cannot hear it as an inner sound. The inner sound is there but it is so silent, so subtle, you don't have the ear to listen to it. The ear has to be developed. When the body and the mind are saturated, only then will you have that ear – the third ear, so to speak – so you can listen to the sound which is always there. It is a cosmic sound. It is in and out. Put your ear to a tree and it is there, put your ear to a rock and it is there. First your body-mind should be transcended, and you should gain more and more energy. The subtle will require tremendous energy to be heard.

With the first step sex disappears, with the second step love disappears, and with the third step everything that you have known disappears – as if you are no more, dead, gone, dissolved. It is a death phenomenon.

If you don't become scared and escape... And the tendency will be to escape, because this looks like an abyss and you are falling into it, and it is bottomless. There seems to be no end to it. You become like a feather falling into a bottomless abyss – falling and falling and falling, and there seems to be no end to it. You will become scared. You would like to run away. If you run away from it, the whole effort you have made would have been a wastage. If you start running, the first thing to do is to begin chanting the mantra om because if you chant you are back in the mind. And if you chant loudly you are back in the body.

So when one starts listening, one shouldn't chant because it will be an escape. A mantra has to be chanted and dropped. A mantra is complete only when you can drop it. If you go on chanting it you will cling to it like a shelter, and whenever you become afraid you will again chant it.

That's why I say, "Chant it so deeply that the body is saturated." There is no need to chant in the body again. The mind is saturated, overflowing, so there is no need to chant it, there is no space to put more chanting into it. So you cannot escape. Only then the soundless sound becomes possible.

Another friend has asked:

Osho,
Before, you used to talk about the mantra *hoo*. Why are you now emphasizing the mantra om?

I am not emphasizing; I am simply explaining Patanjali to you. My emphasis remains with *hoo*. And whatever I am saying about om, the same is applicable to *hoo*. But my emphasis remains with *hoo*.

As I told you, Patanjali existed five thousand years ago. People were simple – very simple and innocent. They could trust easily; they were not so much in the mind. They were not head oriented; they were heart oriented. Om is a mild sound – soothing, nonviolent, nonaggressive. So if you chant om, it goes from the throat to the heart, never below it. Those were heart people. Om was enough for them – a mild dose, a homeopathic dose was enough for them.

For you, it won't help much. For you, *hoo* will be more helpful. *Hoo* is a Sufi mantra; just as om is a Hindu mantra. *Hoo* is a Mohammedan, Sufi mantra, and was developed by Sufis for a very aggressive, violent country and race; not simple, innocent people, but cunning and clever fighters. *Hoo* was invented for them.

Hoo is the last part of Allah. If you repeat "Allah, Allah, Allah, Allah" continuously, by and by it takes the shape of "*Allahoo, Allahoo, Allahoo.*" By and by, the first part is dropped. It becomes "*Lahoo, lahoo, lahoo.*" Then even the "ah" is dropped. It becomes "*Hoo, hoo, hoo.*" It is very forceful, and it directly hits your sex center. It doesn't hit your heart, it hits your sex center.

Hoo will be helpful for you, because now your heart is almost nonfunctioning. Love has disappeared; only sex has remained. Your sex center is functioning, not your love center, so om will not be of much help. *Hoo* will be a deeper help because your energy is not now near the heart. Your energy is near the sex center, and it has to be hit directly so the energy rises upward.

After a period of doing *hoo*, you may feel that you don't need that much of a dose. You can then change over to om. When you start feeling that now you exist near the heart, and not the sex center, only then can you use om – not before it. But there is no need because *hoo* can go the whole way.

You can change if you feel like it. If you feel that now there is no need of chanting *hoo* because you don't feel sexual, are not worried about sex, and don't think about it anymore... If it is not a cerebral imagination, and you are not fascinated by it – a beautiful woman passes by and you simply take a note that yes, a woman has passed, but nothing arises within you, your sex center is not hit, no energy moves in you – then you can start om.

But there is no need to change; you can continue with *hoo*. *Hoo* is a stronger dose. When you chant *hoo*, you can immediately feel that it goes to the stomach – to the hara center – and then to the sex center. It forces the sex energy upward immediately. It stirs the sex center.

You are more head oriented. It always happens that people, countries, civilizations which are head oriented become sexual – more sexual than heart oriented people. Heart oriented people are loving. Sex comes as a shadow of love; it is not important in itself. Heart oriented people don't think about it much, but really, if you watch, twenty-three, twenty-four hours, you are thinking about sex.

Heart oriented people don't think about sex at all. When it happens, it happens. It is just like a body need. And it follows as a shadow to love; it never happens directly. They live in the middle – the heart is the middle between the head and the sex centers. You live in the head and in the sex. You move from these two extremes; you are never in the middle. When sex is fulfilled, you move to the heart; when the desire for sex arises you move to sex. But you never stay in the middle. The pendulum moves right and left – never stops in the middle.

Patanjali developed this method of chanting om for very simple people, innocent villagers living with nature. You can try it; if it helps, it is good. But my understanding about you is that it will not help more than one percent of you. Ninety-nine percent will be helped by the mantra *hoo*. It is nearer to you.

And remember, when the mantra *hoo* succeeds, when you reach the listening point, you will listen to *omkar*, not *hoo*; you will listen to om. The final phenomenon will be the same. *Hoo* is just on the path. You are difficult people! Stronger doses are needed, that's all. But on the final step, you will experience the same phenomenon.

My emphasis remains with *hoo* because my emphasis does not depend on Hindus or Mohammedans; my emphasis depends on you, what your need is. I am neither a Hindu nor a Mohammedan; I am nobody, so I am free. I can use anything from anywhere. A Hindu will feel guilty using Allah; a Mohammedan will feel guilty using om. But I am not fussy about such things. If Allah helps, it is beautiful; if *omkar* helps, it is beautiful. I bring every method to you according to your need.

To me, all religions lead to the same; the goal is one. All religions are like paths leading to the same summit. On the top, everything becomes one. Now it depends on you – where you are, and which path will be nearer. Om will be very far from you; *hoo* is much nearer. It is your need. My emphasis depends on your need. My emphasis is not theoretical, it is not sectarian; my emphasis is absolutely personal. I look at you and decide.

The fourth question:

Osho,
You said that needs are to do with the body and desires
are to do with the mind. Which of these two brought us
to you?

Before I answer this, one more thing has to be understood; it will then be possible for you to understand the answer to this question. You are not only the body and mind; you are something else also – the soul, the self, the atman. The body has needs, the atman also has needs; just between the two is the mind which has desires. The body has needs – hunger and thirst to be satisfied. Shelter, food, water is needed. The body has needs; the mind has desires. Nothing is needed, but the mind creates false needs. A desire is a false need. If you don't attend to it you feel frustrated, a failure. If you attend to it, nothing is attained because in the first place it was never a need, it never existed as a need.

You can fulfill a need; you cannot fulfill a desire. Desire is a dream. A dream cannot be fulfilled; it has no roots, neither in the earth, nor in the sky. It has no roots. Mind is a dreaming phenomenon. You ask for fame, name, prestige. Even if you attain them you will not attain anything because fame will not satisfy any need. It is not a need. You may become famous. If the whole earth knows about you, what then? What will happen to you? What can you do with it? It is neither food nor drink. When the whole world knows you, you will feel frustrated. What to do with it? It is useless.

The soul again has needs. Just as the body has a need for food, the soul also has a need for food. Of course, the food is God. You must remember Jesus saying to his disciples many times, "Eat me, I am your food. And let me be your drink." What does he mean? It is a different need. Unless it is satisfied, unless you can eat God, unless you become God by eating him, absorbing him so that he flows in your soul like blood and becomes your consciousness, you will remain unsatisfied.

The soul has needs, and religion fulfills those needs. The body has needs; science fulfills those needs. The mind has desires and tries to fulfill them, but cannot. It is just a boundary line where body and soul meet. When body and soul are separate, the mind simply disappears. It has no existence of its own.

Now take this question: "You said that needs are to do with the body and desires are to do with the mind. Which of these two brought us to you?"

There are three types of people around me: one group have come because of their body needs. They are frustrated with sex, frustrated with love, miserable in the body. They have come, and they can be helped; their problem is honest, and once their body needs disappear, their soul needs will arise.

The second group have come because of their soul needs. They can be helped because they have real needs. They have not come for their sex problems, love problems, body diseases, or illnesses. They have not come for that. They have come to seek the truth; they have come to enter the mystery of life; they have come to know what existence is.

Then there is a third group – this group is greater than both the other two. They have come because of their mind desires. They cannot be helped. They will hang around me for some time and disappear. Or, if they hang around me for a longer time, I may reduce them to either body needs or soul needs, but their mind needs cannot be fulfilled because they are not needs in the first place.

There are a few people who are here for egoistic reasons. Sannyas is an ego trip for them. They become special, extraordinary. They have failed in life: they couldn't attain political power, they couldn't reach worldly fame, they couldn't achieve wealth, material things. They feel like they are nobodies. I give them sannyas, and without doing anything on their part, they become somebody important, special. Just by changing to orange clothes, now they think they are not ordinary people, they are the chosen few – different from everybody else. They will go into the world and condemn everybody: "You are just worldly creatures. You are absolutely wrong and doomed. We are the saved ones, the chosen few."

These are mind desires. Remember not to be here for any mind desire; otherwise you are simply wasting your time. They cannot be fulfilled. I am here to bring you out of your dreams, I am not here to fulfill your dreams. These people will bring all types of politics here because they are on an ego trip. They will bring all sorts of conflicts; they will create cliques. They will create a miniature world here, and they will create a hierarchy: "I am higher than you, holier than you." They will play the game of one-upmanship.

They are fools. They should not be here in the first place. They have chosen the wrong place for their ego trips because I am here to completely kill their egos, to shatter them. That's why you feel so much chaos around me. Remember, you can be in the right place for the wrong reasons; then you miss, because the question is not the place, the question is why you are here. If you are here for your body needs, something can be done, and when your body needs are settled, your soul needs will arise.

If you are here for your mind needs, drop them. They are not needs, they are dreams. Drop them as completely as is possible. And don't ask how to drop them because nothing is needed to be done in order for them to drop. Just the very understanding that they are mind desires is enough – they drop automatically.

The fifth question:

Osho,
Is it possible to find a synthesis between Yoga and
Tantra? Does one lead to the other?

No, it is impossible. It is as impossible as if you would try to
find a synthesis between man and woman.

What will be the synthesis? – a third sex; an impotent person
will be the synthesis, and that will be neither man nor woman.
That man will be nowhere, rootless.

Tantra is the absolute opposite, diametrically opposite to
Yoga. You cannot make any synthesis. And never try such things
because you will be more and more confused. One is enough to
confuse you; two will be too much – they lead in different directions. They reach the same summit, they reach the same peak.
Synthesis is there at the top, at the climax, but at the foothill,
where the journey starts, they are absolutely different. One goes
to the east, another goes to the west. They say good-bye to each
other; they have their backs to each other. They are like man and
woman – different psychologies, beautiful in their difference.

If you make a synthesis, it becomes ugly. A woman has to be
a woman, so much of a woman that she becomes a polarity
to man. In their polarities they are beautiful because they are
attracted to each other. In their polarities they are complemen-
tary, but you cannot synthesize. Synthesis will just be poor, and it
will be powerless. There will be no tension in it. They meet at the
peak, and that meeting is orgasm. Where man and woman meet,
when their bodies dissolve, when they are not two things, when
both yin and yang are one, it becomes one circle of energy. For a
moment, at the summit of their bioenergy they meet, and fall
back down again.

It is the same with Tantra and Yoga. Tantra is feminine, Yoga
is male; Tantra is surrender, Yoga is will. Tantra is effortlessness,
Yoga is effort – tremendous effort. Tantra is passive, Yoga is
active. Tantra is like the earth, Yoga is like the sky. They meet,

but there is no synthesis. They meet at the top, but at the foothill where the journey starts, where you are all standing, you have to choose the path.

Paths cannot be synthesized, and people who try that confuse humanity. The confusion is very deep, and they are not helpful, they are very harmful. Paths cannot be synthesized, only the end. One path has to be separate from another path – perfectly separate, different in its very tone, its very being. When you follow Tantra you move through sex. And that is Tantra's path; you allow nature a total surrender. It is a let-go – you don't fight; it is not a path of a warrior. You don't struggle; you surrender to wherever nature leads. Nature leads into sex, you surrender to sex. You completely move into it with no guilt, with no concept of sin.

Tantra has no concept of sin, no guilt. Move into sex. Just remain alert, watching what is happening. Be alert, mindful of what is going on, but don't try to control it, don't try to contain yourself; allow the flow. Move into the woman, let the woman move into you. Let yourselves become a circle and remain the watcher. Through this watching and let-go, Tantra achieves a transcendence; sex disappears. This is one way to go beyond nature because going beyond sex is going beyond nature.

The whole of nature is sexual. Flowers bloom because they are sexual. All beauty exists because of some sexual phenomenon. A continuous game is going on. Trees are attracting other trees, birds are calling to others; a sexual game is going on everywhere. Nature is sex, and to achieve to supersex is to go beyond sex. But Tantra says, "Use sex as a step." Don't fight it; go beyond it by using it. Move through it, pass through it, and attain the transcendence through experience. A watchful experience becomes transcendence.

Yoga says, "Don't waste energy; bypass sex completely." No need to go into it, you can simply bypass it. Conserve energy, and don't be fooled by nature. Fight nature, and become a willpower; become a controlled being not floating anywhere. The whole of Yoga, its methods, are how to make you capable so that there is no need to let go into nature, no need to allow nature to have its own way. You become a master and move on your own against nature, fighting nature. It is the way of the warrior, the impeccable warrior who continuously fights, and through fighting transcends.

These two paths are totally different, and both lead to the same goal. Choose one, and don't try to synthesize. How can you synthesize? If you go through sex, Yoga is dropped. If you leave sex, Tantra is dropped. But remember, both lead to the same goal – transcendence is the goal. It depends on you, on your type. Are you the warrior type, a man who fights continuously? – Yoga is your path. If you are not the warrior type, if you are passive, in a subtle way feminine; if you don't like fighting with anyone, and are really nonviolent, Tantra is the path. There is no need to synthesize because both lead to the same goal.

To me, the synthesizers are almost always wrong. All Gandhis are wrong. Whoever synthesizes is wrong – it is synthesizing allopathy with ayurvedic, it is synthesizing homeopathy with allopathic, it is synthesizing Hindu with Mohammedan, it is synthesizing Buddha and Patanjali.

Each path is perfect in itself, there is no need to synthesize. Each path is so perfect in itself that it doesn't need anything added to it. Any addition can be dangerous because a part which may be functioning in a particular machine may become a barrier in another.

You can take a part from an Impala car, which was functioning well in it, and you can put it in a Ford and it may create problems. A part functions in a pattern, a part depends on the pattern, on the whole. You simply cannot use a part anywhere. And what do these synthesizers do? – they take a part from one system, another part from another system, and make a hotchpotch. If you follow these fellows you will become a hotchpotch. No need to synthesize. Just try to find out what type you are, feel your type – and there is no hurry; watch and feel your type.

Can you surrender, surrender to nature? – then surrender. If you feel it is impossible, "I cannot surrender," don't be depressed. There is another path which needs no surrender in this way, which gives you the opening to fight. Both lead to the same at the peak, when you have reached Gourishankar. By and by, as you reach nearer and nearer to the peak, you see others who are also reaching it, and they were traveling on different paths.

Ramakrishna tried one of the greatest experiments in the whole history of humanity. After he became enlightened, he tried many paths. Nobody has ever done that because there is no need. You have attained the peak; why be worried whether other paths lead to it or not? But Ramakrishna did a great service to humanity. He came back down to the foothill again and tried another path to find out whether it also leads to the top or not. He tried many, and each time he reached the same point.

This is his metaphor: that at the foothill paths are different, they move in different directions – they even look opposite, contradictory – but at the top they meet. Synthesis is at the top. In the beginning there are diversions, multiplicity; in the end unity, oneness.

Don't bother about synthesis. Simply choose your path and stick to it. And don't be allured by others who will be calling you to come to their path because it leads… Hindus, Mohammedans, Jews, Christians have all reached. And for the ultimate truth there is no conditioning that you will only reach if you are a Hindu.

The only thing to be worried about is to feel your type and to choose. I am not against anything; I am for everything. Whatever you choose, I can help you that way. But no synthesis – don't try for the synthesis.

The sixth question:

Osho,
Often when you are talking to us, waves of energy come

opening our hearts and bringing tears of gratitude. You
have said that you fill us whenever we are open, but
often this phenomenon happens to many people at the
same time, like *shaktipat*. Why don't you give us this
wonderful experience more often?

It is up to you; it's not that I am giving you any experience.
It is up to you if you take the experience. It is not a giving
because I am giving all the time. It is for you to be open and take
it. And it is right that it happens many times to many people at
the same time. The logical mind says that I must be doing something; otherwise, why is it happening to so many people at the
same time?

No, I am not doing anything. But when one opens, the opening
of that one is infectious, and immediately others start opening. It is
just like when one person starts coughing and then others start; it
is infectious. One person opens, and suddenly you feel something is
happening all around; you also become open.

I am continuously available. Whenever you open you can
share me, whenever you are closed, you cannot share. It is not
up to me; it is up to you to do something. Of course, it happens
all together because one opens another, and it goes on and on. It
can become a floodlike phenomenon.

In Indonesia there is a particular method known as *latihan*.
They use the word *opening*: one who is open can open others.
The master is a man called Bapak Subud. He is one of the most
significant men upon this earth right now; he is the master of
latihan. He has opened a few people, and he tells them to go
around the earth and open others.

What do they do? – they do a very simple method. You will
be able to understand it because you are doing many methods on
similar lines here. One who is opened by Bapak Subud moves
with a newcomer – one who is to be opened, the disciple. They
stand in a closed room. The one who is already open raises his

hands toward the sky. He opens himself, and the other simply stands there. Within a few minutes the other starts trembling. Something is happening, and when he is opened – opened to the infinite sky, to the infinite energy from the beyond – he is then allowed to open others.

Nobody knows what they do; even the doer never knows what he is doing. He simply stands there and the other, the neophyte, just stands nearby, and neither of them know. They ask Bapak Subud, "What is this?" They do it – it happens – but Bapak Subud never gives any explanation. He is not that type of man. He says, "Simply do it. Don't bother why it happens – it happens!"

The same happens here. One opens, and suddenly the energy moves around him; he creates a milieu. If you are near him, suddenly you feel a surge rising up, tears start flowing, your heart is full. You open, you help another... It becomes a chain reaction. The whole world can be opened, and once you are open you know the knack of it. It is not a method, you simply know the knack of it. You simply put your mind in a certain situation, your being in a certain way. This is what I call prayer.

To me, prayer is not a verbal communication to the divine because how can you communicate in language with the divine? The divine has no language – whatever you say will not be understood. You can be understood not by language, but by your being. The being is the only language.

Try this small prayer method: at night time, when you are going to bed, just kneel down near the bed. Put the light off, raise both your hands, close your eyes, and feel as if you are under a waterfall – an energy waterfall from the sky. In the beginning it is imagination; in the beginning it has to be imagination. Within two or three days you start feeling that it is a real phenomenon – that you are under a waterfall. Your body starts shaking as if it is a leaf in a strong wind. And the fall is so strong and tremendous you cannot contain it; it fills your every pore, from toe to head.

You have become just an empty vessel and it fills you.

When you feel trembling arising in you, cooperate with it. Help the trembling to grow more because the more you tremble, the more the possibility is for the infinite energy to descend in you – because your own inner energy becomes dynamic. When you are dynamic, you can meet the dynamic force; when you are static, you cannot meet the dynamic force. When you tremble, energy is created within you. Energy attracts more energy. Become a vessel – filled, overflowing. When you feel that now it is too much, unbearable, that the fall is coming nearer and you cannot bear it any longer, bow down to the earth, kiss the earth and remain there silent, as if you are pouring the energy into the earth.

Take from the sky, give back to the earth. You become just a medium in between. Bow down completely, become empty again. When you feel you are now empty, you will feel so silent, calm, collected. Raise your hands again, let yourself fill up with the energy. Go down, kiss the earth, and give the energy back to the earth.

Energy is sky, energy is earth. There are two types of energy: the sky is always called the male because it gives, and the earth is always called the female because it takes, it is like a womb. So take from the sky and give to the earth. This has to be done seven times, not less, because each time the energy will penetrate one chakra of your body, and there are seven chakras.

Each time the energy will go deeper in you; it will stir a deeper core within you. Seven times is a must. You should not do less because if you do less you will not be able to sleep. The energy will be inside and you will feel restless. Do it seven times. You can do more, there is no harm in it, but not less. Do it seven times or more. When you feel completely empty, go to sleep. The whole night will become a happening. In your sleep you will become more and more silent. Dreams will stop. In the morning you will feel a completely new being arising, resurrected. You are no longer the old; the past has dropped, you are fresh and young.

Do it every night. Within three months many things will become possible. You will be open, and you can open others. After doing this opening phenomenon for three months, you can simply stand by the side of someone and open yourself, and immediately you will feel that the other is shaking, trembling. Even if he doesn't know it, even without his knowing you can open someone. But don't do that because the other will be scared. He will think that something weird is happening.

Once opened, you can open others. It is an infection, and a beautiful infection; an infection of perfect health, not of any disease – an infection of wholeness, holiness, infection of the sacred.

Enough for today.

9

How to Become More Beautiful and Happy

The mind becomes tranquil by cultivating attitudes of friendliness toward the happy, compassion toward the miserable, joy toward the virtuous and indifference toward the evil.

The mind also becomes tranquil by alternately expelling and retaining the breath.

When meditation produces extraordinary sense perceptions, the mind gains confidence and this helps perseverance.

Also, meditate on the inner light which is serene and beyond all sorrow.

Also, meditate on one who has attained desirelessness.

The mind becomes tranquil by cultivating attitudes of friendliness toward the happy, compassion toward the miserable, joy toward the virtuous and indifference toward the evil.

M any things have to be understood before you can understand this sutra. First, the natural attitudes: whenever you see someone happy, you feel jealous – not happy, never happy – you feel miserable. That's the natural attitude, the attitude that you already have. Patanjali says: *The mind becomes tranquil by cultivating attitudes of friendliness toward the happy...* Very difficult. To be friendly with someone who is happy is one of the most difficult things in life. Ordinarily you think it is very easy. It is not! Just the opposite is the case. You feel jealous, you feel miserable. You may show your happiness, but that's just a facade, a show, a mask. If you have such an attitude, how can you be happy? How can you be tranquil, silent?

The whole of life is celebrating; millions of happinesses are happening all over the universe, but if your attitude is of jealousy you will be miserable, you will be in a constant hell. You will be in a hell precisely because all over and around you there is heaven. You will create a hell for yourself, a private hell because the whole of existence is celebrating.

If somebody is happy, what's the first thing that comes to your mind? – it's as if that happiness has been taken from you? As if the person has won and you are defeated? As if he has cheated you? Don't be worried, happiness is not a competition. If somebody is happy, it does not mean that you cannot be happy – that he has taken happiness and now how can you be happy? Happiness does not exist some place where it can be exhausted by happy people.

Why do you feel jealous? If somebody is rich, maybe it is difficult for you to be rich because riches exist in a quantity. If somebody is powerful in a material way, it may be difficult for you to be powerful because power is a competition. But happiness is not a competition. Happiness exists in an infinite quantity. Nobody has ever been able to exhaust it; there is no competition at all. If somebody is happy, why do you feel jealous? And, with jealousy, hell enters you.

Patanjali says, "When somebody is happy, feel happy, feel friendly." Then you also open a door toward happiness. In a subtle way, if you can feel friendly with someone who is happy, you immediately start sharing his happiness; it becomes yours also, immediately! Happiness is not some "thing," it is not material; it is not something that somebody can cling to. You can share it. When a flower blooms you can share it; when a bird sings you can share it; when somebody is happy you can share it. And the beauty is that it does not depend on the person sharing; it depends on your partaking.

It is a totally different thing if it depended on his sharing, on whether he shares or not. He may not like to share. But this is not a question at all, it does not depend on his sharing. When the sun rises in the morning you can be happy, and the sun cannot do anything about it. It cannot prevent you being happy. If somebody is happy, you can be friendly. It is totally your own attitude and he cannot prevent you sharing. You open a door and immediately his happiness flows toward you.

This is the secret of creating a heaven all around you, and only within heaven can you be tranquil. How can you be tranquil in hellfire? And nobody is creating it; you create it. So the basic thing to be understood is that whenever there is misery, hell, you are the cause of it. Never throw the responsibility on anyone else because that throwing of responsibility is escaping from the basic truth. If you are miserable, only you, absolutely only you, are responsible. Look within and find the cause of it. Nobody wants to be miserable. If you can find the cause within you, you can throw it out. Nobody is preventing you by standing in your way. There is not a single obstacle to being happy.

You become attuned to happiness just by being friendly toward happy people. They are flowering, you become friendly. They may not be friendly; that is none of your concern. They may not even know you – that doesn't matter. But wherever there is a blossoming, wherever there is bliss, wherever somebody is flowering, wherever somebody is dancing and is happy and is smiling, wherever there is celebration, you become friendly, you partake of it. It starts flowing within you and nobody can prevent it. When there is happiness all around you, you feel tranquil. *The mind becomes tranquil by cultivating attitudes of friendliness toward the happy...*

With the happy you feel jealous – in a subtle competition. You feel inferior with happy people. You always choose to have people around you who are unhappy. You become friendly with unhappy people because with them you feel superior. You always seek somebody who is below you. You are afraid of the higher; you always seek the lower, and the more you seek the lower, the lower you fall. Then even lower people are needed.

Seek the company of those who are higher than you – higher in wisdom, happiness, tranquillity, calmness, quietness, collectedness. Always seek the company of the higher because that is the way you become higher, and how you transcend the valleys and reach to the peaks. That becomes a ladder. Always seek the company of the higher, the beautiful, the happy, and you will become more beautiful and happy.

Once the secret is known, once you know how one becomes happier, and how with others' happiness you create a situation for yourself to be happy, there is no barrier; you can go as far as you like. You can become a god where no unhappiness exists.

Who is a god? – he is one who has learned the secret of being happy with the whole universe, with every flower, river, rock and star; who has become one with this continuous eternal celebration; who celebrates, and who doesn't bother whose celebration this is. Wherever there is a celebration, he participates. This art of participating in happiness is one of the foundations if you want happiness. It has to be followed.

You have been doing just the opposite. If somebody is happy, immediately you are shocked – how is it possible? How come you're not happy and he is? There is injustice. This whole world is cheating you and there is no God. If God is, how come you are not happy and others are? And these people who are happy, they are the exploiters, they are tricky, cunning. They live on your blood. They are sucking others' happiness.

Nobody is sucking anybody's happiness. Happiness is such a phenomenon that there is no need to suck it. It's an inner flowering; it doesn't come from the outside. Just by being happy with happy people, you create the situation in which your own inner flower starts blossoming. *The mind becomes tranquil by cultivating attitudes of friendliness...*

You create enmity. You feel friendly with a sad person and you think it's virtuous. You can feel friendly with someone who is depressed, in misery, and you think it is something religious, that you are doing something moral – you don't know what you're doing.

Whenever you feel friendly with someone who is sad or depressed, unhappy, miserable, you create misery for yourself. Patanjali's attitude looks very irreligious. It is not, because when you understand his whole standpoint you will see what he means. He is very scientific. He is not a sentimental person, and sentimentality won't help you. One has to be very, very clear.

...compassion toward the miserable... Not friendliness – compassion. Compassion is a different quality to friendliness.

Friendliness means you are creating a situation in which you would like to be the same as the other person – you would like to be the same as your friend. Compassion means that someone has fallen from his state. You would like to help him, but you would not like to be like him. You would like to give him a hand; you would like to bring him up, cheer him up. You would like to help him in every way, but you would not like to be like him because that is not a help.

If somebody is crying and weeping, and you sit by their side and start crying and weeping too, are you helping him? In what way? If somebody is miserable and you become miserable, are you helping him? You may be doubling his misery. He was miserable alone; now there are two miserable people. But in showing sympathy to the miserable you are again playing a trick. Deep down, when you show sympathy to the miserable – and remember, sympathy is not compassion; sympathy is friendliness – when you show sympathy and friendliness to a depressed, sad, miserable person, deep down you are feeling happy. There is always an undercurrent of happiness.

It has to be so because it is simple arithmetic. When someone is happy, you feel miserable – so how is it possible that when somebody is miserable you can feel unhappy? If when somebody is happy you feel miserable, then when somebody is unhappy, deep down you feel very happy. But you don't show it. Or, if you are acutely observed you show it; even in your sympathy there is a subtle current of happiness. You feel good and really cheered up, that it is not you who is unhappy and that you are in a position to show sympathy – you are higher, superior.

People always feel good when they have the opportunity to show sympathy to others; they are always cheered by it. Deep down they feel that they are not so miserable, thank God! When somebody dies, immediately an undercurrent in you thanks God that you are still alive, and can show sympathy, and it costs nothing. Showing sympathy costs nothing, but compassion is a different thing. Compassion means you would like to help the other person; you would like to do whatever can be done; you would like to help him to come out of his misery. You are not happy about it, but you are also not miserable. Compassion exists just between the two.

Buddha is in compassion. He will not feel miserable with you because that is not going to help anyone, and he will not feel happy because there is no point in feeling happy. How can you feel happy when somebody is miserable? But he cannot feel unhappy either because that is not going to help. He will feel compassion. And compassion exists just in between these two. Compassion means he would like to help you to come out of it. Compassion means he is for you, but against your misery; he loves you, but not your misery. He would like to bring you up – but not with your misery.

When you are sympathetic you start loving the misery, not the man who is miserable. If suddenly the man cheers up and says, "Don't bother," you will feel shocked because he never gave you a chance to be sympathetic and show him how much higher, superior and happier a being you are.

Don't be miserable with somebody who is miserable. Help him to come out of it. Never make misery an object of love; don't give any affection to misery because if you give affection and make it an object of love you are opening a door for it. Sooner or later you will become miserable. Remain aloof. Compassion means, remain aloof. Extend your hand, remain aloof, help – don't feel miserable, don't feel happy because both are the same. On the surface, when you feel miserable with somebody's misery, deep down is the current of being happy. Both have to be dropped. Compassion will bring you tranquillity of the mind.

Many people come to me – social reformers, revolutionaries, politicians, utopians, and say, "How can you teach people meditation and silence when there is so much misery in the world? This is selfish." They would like me to teach people to be miserable together with others who are miserable. They don't know what they are saying, but they feel very good – doing social work, social service, they feel very good. If suddenly the world becomes a heaven, and God says, "Now everything will be okay," you will find social reformers and revolutionaries in absolute misery because they will have nothing to do.

Kahlil Gibran has written a small parable:

In a big city, there was a dog who was a preacher and missionary, and preached to other dogs, "Stop barking! We are wasting almost ninety-nine percent of our energy in unnecessarily barking. That's why we have not been evolving. Stop barking unnecessarily!"

But it is difficult for dogs to stop barking. That is an inbuilt process. Really, they only feel happy when they bark. It is a catharsis. They feel silent after they have barked. So they listened to the leader, the revolutionary, the utopian who was thinking somewhere in the coming future of a kingdom of gods, a kingdom of dogs. A kingdom where every dog is reformed and has become religious – where there is no barking, no fighting, where everything is silent. That missionary must have been a pacifist.

But dogs are dogs. They would listen to him and say, "You are a great man, and whatever you say is true, but we are helpless, poor dogs. We don't understand such big things." So all the dogs felt guilty because they couldn't stop. They believed in the message of the leader, and he was right. They could follow rationally, but what to do with their bodies? Their bodies are irrational. Whenever there is a chance – a sannyasin walking by, a policeman, a postman, they bark because they are against uniforms.

It was almost impossible for them, and they had all agreed: "That dog is a great man, and we cannot follow him. He is like an avatar – something from the other shore – so we will worship him, but how can we follow him?" And that leader was true to his word, he never barked. But one day everything failed. One dark night the dogs decided: "This great leader is always trying to convert us, and we never listen to him. At least once a year, on his birthday, we should keep a complete fast with no barking, absolute silence, no matter how difficult. At least once a year we will do that."

And on that night not a single dog barked. The leader watched from this corner to that, from this street to that because wherever dogs are barking he would start to preach. He started feeling very miserable because nobody was barking; the whole night was completely silent, as if no dog existed. He went to many places, watched, and by midnight it became impossible for him; he walked into a dark corner and barked!

The moment the other dogs heard that one dog had broken the silence, they said, "Now there's no problem." They didn't know that the leader had done it; they thought one of them had broken the vow. But now it was impossible for them to contain themselves – the whole city barked. The leader came out and started preaching!

This is the condition of your social revolutionaries, reformers, Gandhians, Marxists and others – all brands. They will be in great difficulty if the world is really changed. If the world really fulfills the utopia of their minds and imagination, they will commit suicide or they will go mad. Or they will just start preaching the contradictory, the opposite of whatever they are preaching now.

They come to me and say, "How can you tell people to be silent when the world is in such misery?" They think that first the misery has to be removed, and then people will be silent? No, if people are silent misery can be removed because only silence can remove the misery. Misery is an attitude. It is less concerned with material conditions, more concerned with the inner mind, the inner consciousness. Even a poor man can be happy, and once he is happy many things start falling in line.

Soon he may not be a poor man because how can you be poor when you are happy? When you are happy, the whole world participates with you. When you are unhappy, everything goes wrong. You create a situation all around which helps your unhappiness to exist. This is the dynamics of the mind. It is a self-defeating system. You feel miserable, then more misery is attracted to you. When more misery is attracted you say, "How can I be silent? There is so much misery." Then even more misery is attracted toward you. When you have attracted more misery you say, "It's impossible now. Those people who say they are happy must be telling lies; These Buddhas, Krishnas, must be telling lies. These Patanjalis must be liars because how's it possible to be happy when there is so much misery?"

You are in a self-defeating system. You attract misery, and you attract it not only for yourself; when one person is miserable, he helps others to be miserable too because they are also fools like you. Seeing you in misery, they sympathize. When they sympathize they become vulnerable. So it is just like that – one sick person infects the whole community.

Mulla Nasruddin's small son was ill. His doctor sent him a bill. It was too much, so Nasruddin phoned the doctor.

"This is too much."

The doctor replied, "But I had to come nine times to see your son, so that has to be accounted for."

Nasruddin said, "Don't forget that my son infected the whole village and you have been earning a lot from that. In fact, you should pay me something."

When one person is miserable, he infects other people. Misery is infectious, just as happiness is infectious. As you are, you are vulnerable to misery because you are always seeking it unknowingly; your mind seeks misery because with misery you feel sympathy; with happiness you feel jealousy.

Mulla Nasruddin's wife once asked me, "If you are going to

New Delhi – the winter is coming – will you bring me a drop-dead coat?"

I was surprised. I couldn't follow what she meant. I said to her, "I don't know much about coats, but I have never heard... What is a drop-dead coat?"

She replied, "You haven't heard of it?" She started laughing and said, "A drop-dead coat is a coat which when you put it on, the neighbors drop dead!"

Unless others drop dead you don't feel alive. Unless others are miserable you don't feel happy. But how can you feel happy when others are unhappy, and how can you feel really alive when others are dead? We exist together.

Sometimes you may be the cause of many people's misery – then you are earning karma. You may not have directly hit them, you may not have been violent to them. The law is subtle. You need not be a murderer, but if you simply infect people with your misery, you are participating in it; you are creating misery. You are responsible for it, and you will have to pay for it. The mechanism is very subtle!

Just two, three days ago a sannyasin attacked Laxmi. You may not have observed the fact that you all are responsible for it because many of you have been feeling antagonistic toward Laxmi. That sannyasin is just a victim, the weakest link among you. He has expressed your antagonism, that's all, and he was the weakest. He became the victim, and now you will feel that he is responsible. That's not true – you participated. The law is subtle...

How have you participated in it? – Laxmi is managing things around here, and deep down whenever somebody is in that role, there are many situations in which you will feel antagonistic towards her; situations in which she will have to say no to you, and you will feel hurt. It cannot be avoided. There are many situations in which you feel that not enough attention is being paid to you, in which you feel that you are treated as a nobody. Your ego feels hurt and you feel antagonistic.

If many people feel antagonistic toward a person, the weakest amongst them will become the victim; he will do something. He was the craziest amongst you, that's right, but he alone is not responsible. If you have ever felt any antagonism toward Laxmi, that is your part and you have earned a karma; unless you become so subtly aware you cannot become enlightened. Things are very complicated.

Now, in the West psychoanalysts have also found that if one person goes mad, the whole family is responsible – the whole family! Now they think that the whole family has to be treated, not one person because when one person goes mad that only shows that the whole family has inner tensions. He is the weakest of them all, so immediately he shows the whole thing; he becomes the expression of the whole family, and if you treat him it won't help. In the hospital he may be okay, back at home he will fall ill again because the whole family has inner tensions and he is the weakest person.

Children suffer far too much because of the parents – they fight, and are always creating anxiety and tension around the house. The whole house exists not as a peaceful community but as an inner war and conflict. The child is more vulnerable; the child starts behaving in eccentric ways – now you have an excuse that you are tense and worried because of the child. Now the father and mother can be concerned with the child; they will take him to a psychoanalyst and a doctor, and they can forget their own conflict.

This child becomes a cementing force. If he is ill, they have to pay more attention to him. Now they have an excuse for why they are worried and tense and in anguish – because the child is ill. They don't know that the reverse is the case, that it is because they are worried, tense, and in conflict. The child is innocent, tender; he can be affected immediately, he has no protection around him yet. And if the child becomes really healthy, the parents will be in more difficulty because then there is no excuse.

This is a community; you live here as a family. Many tensions are bound to exist – be aware. Be alert about those tensions because they can create a force. They can become accumulative, and suddenly somebody who is weak, vulnerable, simple, may become the shelter of the accumulated force, and he reacts. You can then all throw the responsibility on him. But that's not right. If you have ever felt any antagonism, you are part of it. And the same is also true in the greater world.

When Godse murdered Gandhi, I never felt that he was responsible. He was the weakest link, that is true, but the whole of the Hindu mind was responsible – deep currents of Hindu antagonism against Gandhi. The feeling was accumulating that Gandhi was for Muslims, Mohammedans. This is an actual phenomenon, and antagonism accumulates. It hovers just like a cloud and then somewhere a weak heart, an unprotected man, becomes the victim. The cloud gets its roots in him and then the explosion. And everybody is freed; Godse is responsible for murdering Gandhi, so you can kill Godse and be finished with it. The whole country moves in the same way, and the Hindu mind remains the same – no change. The law is subtle.

Always find the dynamics of the mind. Only then will you be transformed; otherwise not. *The mind becomes tranquil by cultivating attitudes of friendliness toward the happy, compassion toward the miserable, joy toward the virtuous…*

Look! Patanjali is making steps – beautiful and very subtle, but exactly scientific. *…joy toward the virtuous, and indifference toward the evil.* When you feel somebody is a virtuous man – joy. The ordinary attitude is that he must be deceiving you. How can anybody be more virtuous than you? Hence so much criticism goes on.

Whenever somebody is virtuous you immediately start criticizing and finding fault with him. Somehow or other you have to bring him down. He cannot be virtuous. You cannot believe this.

Patanjali says *joy* because if you criticize a virtuous man, deep down you are criticizing virtue. If you criticize a virtuous man, you are coming to a point in believing that virtue is impossible in this world. Then you will feel at ease. You can easily move in your evil ways because you feel that nobody is virtuous: "Everybody is just like me – even worse than me." That's why so much condemnation goes on – criticism and condemnation.

If somebody says, "That person is very beautiful," you immediately find something to criticize about. You can't tolerate it because if somebody is virtuous and you are not, your ego is shattered, and you start feeling, "I have to change myself," which is an arduous effort. The simplest way is to condemn, the simplest way is to criticize, the simplest way is to say, "No! Prove what are you saying? First, prove how he is virtuous!" It is difficult to prove virtue. It is very easy to disprove anything; it is very difficult to prove.

Turgenev is one of the greatest Russian storytellers. He has written a story:

In a small village there was a man who was thought to be stupid, and he was; the whole town laughed at him. He was just like a fool, and everybody enjoyed his foolishness. But he was tired of his foolishness, so he asked a wise man, "What should I do?"

The wise man replied, "Nothing! Whenever someone is praising someone else, you simply condemn him. When somebody says, 'That man is a saint,' immediately say, 'No! I know very well that he is a sinner!' Or if somebody says, 'This book is great,' immediately say, 'I have read and studied it.' Don't bother whether you have read it or not; simply say, 'The book is rubbish.' If somebody says, 'This painting is one of the greatest works of art,' simply say, 'But what is it? – just a canvas and colors. A child can do it!' Criticize, say no, ask for proof, and come back to me after seven days."

Within seven days the town started feeling that the man was a genius: "We never knew about his talents, and he is a genius about everything. You show him a painting and he shows you the faults. You show him a great book and he shows the faults. He has such a great critical mind – an analyst, a genius!"

On the seventh day he came back to the wise man and said, "Now there is no need for me to take any advice from you. You are a fool!" The whole town used to believe in that sage. They said, "Our genius has said that he is a fool. So he must be."

People easily believe in the negative because to disprove a no is very difficult – how can you prove it? How can you prove that Jesus is the son of God? How will you prove it? Two thousand years, and Christian theology has been trying to prove it, without success. But within seconds it was proved that he was a sinner, a vagabond, and they killed him – within seconds! Somebody said, "I have seen this man coming out of a prostitute's house" – finished! Nobody bothers whether this man who is saying, "I have seen" is believable or not – nobody bothers. The negative is always easily believed because it is also helping your ego. The positive is not believed.

You can say no whenever there is virtue, but you are not harming the virtuous man, you are harming yourself. You are self-destructive. You are in fact committing suicide slowly, poisoning yourself. When you say, "This man is not virtuous, that man is not virtuous," what are you in fact creating? – you are creating a milieu in which you will come to believe that virtue is impossible; and when virtue is impossible, there is no need to attempt it. You fall down, and settle wherever you are. Growth becomes impossible. You would like to settle, but you will settle in misery because you are miserable. You have all settled completely. This settlement has to be broken; you have to be unsettled. Wherever you are you have to be uprooted and replanted in a higher plane, and that is possible only if you are joyful toward the virtuous.

...joy toward the virtuous and indifference toward the evil.

Don't even condemn evil. The temptation is there; you would even like to condemn virtue, and Patanjali says, "Don't condemn evil." Why? – he knows the inner dynamics of the mind. If you condemn evil too much, and pay too much attention to it, by and by you become attuned to it. If you say that this is wrong, that is wrong, you are paying too much attention to the wrong. You will become addicted to the wrong. If you pay too much attention to anything you become hypnotized. And whatever you are condemning you will commit because it will become an attraction, a deep down attraction. Otherwise, why bother? They are sinners, but who are you to bother about them?

Jesus says, "Judge ye not..." That's what Patanjali means – indifference; don't judge this way or that – be indifferent. Don't say yes or no; don't condemn, don't appreciate. Simply leave it to the divine; it is none of your business. If a man is a thief, it is his business. It is his and God's. Let them settle themselves; you don't come in to it. Who is asking you to come in to it? Jesus says, "Judge ye not"; Patanjali says, "Be indifferent."

One of the greatest hypnotists of the world, Emile Coué, discovered a law – the law of hypnosis. He called it, "The law of reverse effect." If you are too much against something you will become a victim of it. Watch a new person learning to ride a bicycle on the road. The road is sixty feet wide, and there is a milestone by the side of the road. Even if you are a perfect cyclist and you make a target of the stone, "I will go and crash into the stone," sometimes you may miss. But not the new learner – never! He never misses the milestone. In a subtle way his bicycle moves toward the stone, and the road is sixty feet wide! Even with a blindfold you can move toward it – even if there is nobody on the road, it is completely silent, and nobody is moving...

What happens to this new learner? – a law is working; Emile Coué calls it, "The law of reverse effect." Because he is a learner immediately he is afraid, so he looks around for the fear point –

where he can go wrong? The whole of the road is okay, but this stone, this red stone by the corner is the danger. He thinks, "I may crash into it." Now an affinity is created. Now his attention is toward the stone; the whole road is forgotten. And he is a learner. His hands tremble, he is looking at the stone, and by and by he feels that the bicycle is moving...

The bicycle has to follow your attention; the bicycle has no will of its own. It follows you wherever you are going, and you follow your eyes; the eyes follow a subtle hypnosis, an attentiveness. You are looking at the stone so your hands move that way. You become more and more afraid. The more afraid you are, the more you are caught because now the stone seems to be an evil force, as if it is attracting you. The whole road is forgotten, the bicycle is forgotten, the learner is forgotten. Only the stone is there; you are hypnotized. You will crash into the stone. Now you have fulfilled your mind; next time you will be more afraid. Now how to break out of it?

This is what happens when you say that something is wrong. In the monasteries, monks are condemning sex. Sex has become the milestone. They are thinking about it twenty-four hours of the day; trying to avoid it, is thinking about it. The more you try to avoid it, the more you are hypnotized. That is why in the old scriptures it is said that whenever a saint concentrates, beautiful girls from heaven come and try to disturb his mind. Why should beautiful girls be interested in him? Someone is sitting under a tree with closed eyes – why would beautiful girls be interested in him?

Nobody comes from anywhere, but he is so against sex that it becomes a hypnosis. He is so hypnotized that now his dreams become real. He opens his eyes and sees a beautiful naked girl standing before him. You need a pornographic book to see a nude woman. If you go to a monastery you won't need a pornographic book; you create your pornography all around yourself. The seer, the man who was concentrating, becomes more afraid; he closes his eyes, clenches his fist. Now the woman is standing on the inside.

And you cannot find such beautiful women on this earth because they are the creations of dreams, by-products of hypnosis. The more he becomes afraid, the more they are there. They will rub against his body, they will touch his head, cling to and embrace him. He is completely mad, but this does happen. This is also happening to you. Degrees may differ, but this is what is happening. Whatever you are against, deep down you will be joined with it.

Never be against anything. To be against evil is to fall a victim of it. You are falling into the hands of evil. Indifference – if you follow indifference, it means it is none of your concern. If somebody is stealing something, that is his karma; he will know and he will have to suffer. That is not your business at all. Don't think about it, don't pay any attention to it. If somebody is a prostitute, selling her body, that is her business. Don't condemn it, otherwise you will be attracted toward her.

A very old story…

A saint and a prostitute lived together, they were neighbors. The saint was very famous. They both died on the same day.

Death came and started trying to take the saint to hell. The saint was surprised because the prostitute was taken on the road toward heaven. So he said, "What is this? There seems to be some misunderstanding. I am the one who should be led toward heaven – this is a prostitute!"

Death said, "We know, but now if you want we can explain it to you; there is no misunderstanding. These are the orders: the prostitute has to be brought to heaven and the saint has to be thrown into hell."

The saint said, "But why?"

Even the prostitute could not believe it. She said, "Something must be wrong. Must I be thrown in heaven? He is a saint, a great saint. We worshipped him. Take him to heaven."

Death said, "No, that's not possible because he was a saint just on the surface, and he was continuously thinking of you. When you sang in the night, he would come and listen to you. He would stand near the fence and listen to you. And millions of times he would have liked to have come to see you, love you; millions of times he dreamed of you. He was continuously thinking about you. On his lips was the name of God; in his heart was the image of you."

The same was true of the prostitute from the opposite direction. She was selling her body, but always thinking that she would like to have a life like this saint who lives in a temple. "How pure he is!" She dreamed about the saint – the purity, the saintliness, the virtue that she was missing. When her customers had gone, she would pray to God, "Next time don't make me a prostitute again. Make me a worshipper, make me a meditator. I would like to serve in the temple."

Many times she thought about going to the temple, but thought that because she had so much sin, it was not good to enter: "The place is so holy and I am such a sinner." Many times she wanted to touch the feet of the saint, but thought that it would not be good: "I am not worthy enough to touch his feet." So when the saint passed by, she would collect the dust from the road where he had passed, and would worship that dust.

The question is not what you are outwardly. Your future course of life will be decided upon what your inner hypnosis is. Be indifferent to evil. Remember, indifference doesn't mean apathy; these are subtle distinctions. Indifference doesn't mean apathy, it does not mean that you close your eyes, because even if you close them you have taken a standpoint, an attitude. It doesn't mean not to bother because then there is also a subtle condemnation. Indifference simply means: as if it doesn't exist, as if it is not there. Indifference means no attitude. You pass by as if it is not happening.

The word Patanjali uses is very beautiful, *upeksha*. It is neither apathy, antagonism nor escape. It is simple indifference without any attitude – remember, without any attitude because you can be indifferent with an attitude. You can think that it is not worth much – it is not worthy of me to think about it. No, then you have an attitude, and a subtle condemnation is hidden in it. Indifference simply means, who are you to decide, to judge? Think about yourself and ask, "Who are you? How can you say what is evil and what is good? Who knows?"

Life is such a complexity that evil becomes good, good becomes evil – they change. Sinners have been known to reach the ultimate; saints have been known to be thrown into hell. So who knows? And who are you? Who is asking you? Take care of yourself. Even if you can do that, you have done enough. Be more mindful and aware, then an indifference comes to you without any attitude.

It happened...

Vivekananda stayed in the Maharaja of Jaipur's palace before he went to America and became a world famous figure. The Maharaja was a lover of Vivekananda and Ramakrishna. When Vivekananda came to stay in his palace, he made a great festival out of it, and he called on prostitutes to dance and sing in the reception – as maharajas do; they have their own minds. He completely forgot that it doesn't suit the occasion to receive a sannyasin with the singing and dancing of prostitutes. But he didn't know anything else. He knew that when you receive somebody, there was always drinking and dancing.

Vivekananda was still immature; he was not yet a perfect sannyasin. Had he been a perfect sannyasin there would have been indifference – no problem. But he was not indifferent yet; he had not even gone that deep into Patanjali. He was a young man, and a very suppressive one; he was suppressing his sex and everything. When he saw the prostitutes he simply locked himself in his room and wouldn't come out.

The Maharaja came to him and asked his forgiveness. He said, "We didn't know. We have never received sannyasins before. We always receive kings, so we know their ways. We are sorry, but now it will be too insulting because this is the greatest prostitute in the country, and very expensive. We have already paid, so to tell her to move out and leave will be an insult, and if you don't come she will feel very hurt. So come out."

But Vivekananda was afraid to come out; that's why I say that he was still immature, still not a seasoned sannyasin. Indifference was still not there, only a condemnation: "A prostitute?" He was very angry, and said, "No!" The prostitute started singing without him, and she sang a song of a saint. The song is very beautiful. The words of the song are: "I know that I am not worthy of you, but you could have been a little more compassionate. I am dirt on the road, that I know, but you need not be so antagonistic to me. I am nobody, ignorant, a sinner, but you are a saint. Why are you afraid of me?"

It is said that Vivekananda heard the song from his room. The prostitute was weeping and singing, and he became aware of what he was doing. It was immature, childish. Why was he afraid? – fear exists only if you are attracted. You will be afraid of women if you are attracted to them. If you are not attracted, the fear disappears. What is the fear? An indifference comes without any antagonism.

He opened the door. He couldn't contain himself, he was defeated by the prostitute. She was victorious. He had to come out. He came out sat, and wrote in his diary, "A new revelation has been given to me by the divine. I was afraid that it must be some lust within me; that's why I was afraid. But the woman defeated me completely – I have never seen such a pure soul. The tears were so innocent and the singing and the dancing were so holy that I would have missed. Sitting near her, I became aware for the first time that it is not a question of who is there outside; it is a question of what is in."

That night he wrote in his diary, "Now I can even sleep with that woman in the same bed and there will be no fear." He transcended. That prostitute helped him to transcend. This is a miracle. Ramakrishna couldn't help, but a prostitute did.

So nobody knows from where help will come. Nobody knows what is evil and what is good. Who can decide? Mind is impotent and helpless. So don't take any attitude; that is the meaning of being indifferent.

> The mind also becomes tranquil by alternately
> expelling and retaining the breath.

Patanjali also gives other alternatives. If you can do this – being happy with happy people, being friendly; having compassion with the miserable, joy with the virtuous, indifference with the evil ones – you enter from the transformation of the mind toward the supermind. If you cannot – because it is difficult, it is not easy – then there are other ways. Don't feel depressed.

Patanjali says: *The mind also becomes tranquil by alternately expelling and retaining the breath.* You enter through the physiology. The first is entering through the mind; the second is entering through the physiology. Breathing and thinking are deeply connected, as if they are two poles of one thing. You also sometimes become aware, if you are a little mindful, that whenever the mind changes, the breathing changes. For example, if you are angry, immediately your breathing changes, the rhythm is gone. The breathing has a different quality. It is non-rhythmic.

When you have passion, lust, when sex takes over, the breathing changes; it becomes feverish, mad. When you are silent, just not doing anything, just feeling very relaxed, the breathing has a different rhythm. If you watch, and Patanjali must have watched very deeply… He says that if you watch deeply you can find what the type of breathing is, and what type of mind its rhythm creates. If you feel friendly, the breathing is different. If you feel antagonistic, angry, the breathing is different.

So either change the mind and the breathing will change, or you can do the opposite: change the breathing and the mind will change. If you change the rhythm of breathing, the mind will immediately change. When you feel happy, silent, joyous, remember the rhythm of the breathing. Next time when anger comes up, don't allow the breathing to change; retain the rhythm of breathing as if you are happy. Anger is not now possible because the breathing creates the situation. The breathing forces the inner glands of the body to release chemicals in the blood.

That's why you become red when you are angry; certain chemicals come into the blood and you become feverish, your temperature goes high; the body is ready to fight or take flight. The body is in an emergency. Through the hammering of the breathing, this change comes.

Don't change the breathing. Just retain it as if you are silent; the breathing has to follow a silent pattern. You will feel that it is impossible to become angry. When you are feeling very passionate, lustful, sex takes over. Just try to be tranquil with your breathing, and you will feel that sex has disappeared.

Here he suggests a method: *The mind also becomes tranquil by alternately expelling and retaining the breath.* You can do two things. First, whenever you feel that the mind is not tranquil – tense, worried, chattering, in anxiety, constantly dreaming – exhale deeply. Always start by exhaling. Exhale deeply, and throw out as much air as you can. If you throw the air out the mood will also be thrown out because breathing is everything.

And expel the breath as far as possible. Take the belly in and hold it for a few seconds – don't inhale. Let the air out, and don't inhale for a few seconds. Allow the body to inhale. Inhale deeply – as much as you can. Again stop for a few seconds. The gap should be the same as you used when breathing out – if you hold for three seconds, retain the breath for three seconds. Throw it out; hold for three seconds. Inhale, and retain for three seconds. The breath has to be thrown out completely. Exhale totally, inhale totally, and make it a rhythm. Hold, breathe in; retain, breathe out. Hold, in; retain, out. Immediately you will feel a change coming to your whole being. The mood is gone. A new climate has entered you.

What happens? Why is this so? There are many reasons. One, when you start creating this rhythm your mind is completely diverted. You cannot be angry because a new thing has started, and the mind cannot have two things happening together. Your mind is now filled with exhaling, inhaling, retaining, creating a rhythm. You are completely absorbed in it and the cooperation with the anger is broken.

This exhaling and inhaling cleanses the whole body. When you exhale and hold for three or five seconds, or as long as you want, as long as you can, what happens inside? – the whole body throws all that is poisonous into the blood. The air is out, and the body has a gap. In that gap all the poisons are thrown out. They come to the heart and accumulate there – poisonous gases, nitrogen, carbon dioxide; they all gather together there.

Ordinarily, you don't give them a chance to gather together. You go on breathing in and out; there is no gap, no pause in the rhythm. But in that holding, a gap is created, an emptiness. In that emptiness, everything flows and fills it. You take a deep inhalation and retain it. All those poisonous gases become mixed with the breathing; exhale again and throw them out. Again pause, let the poisons gather. This is a way of throwing things out.

The mind and the breath are so very much connected. They have to be because breathing is life. A man can be without a mind, but cannot be without breathing. Breathing is deeper than the mind. Your whole brain can be operated on; you will be alive if you can breathe. If the breathing continues, you will be alive. The brain can be taken out completely. You will vegetate, but you will be alive. You will not be able to open your eyes or talk or do any-thing, but lying on the bed you can stay alive, vegetating for many years. But the mind cannot function without the breath. If the breathing stops, the mind disappears.

Yoga found this basic thing: that breathing is deeper than thinking. If you change the breathing you change the thinking, and once you know the key – that breathing has the key – you can create any climate that you want. It is up to you; it depends on the way you breathe. Do one thing: for seven days, make a note of the different types of breathing that happen with your different moods. When you are angry, count your breathing and make a note – how much you inhale and how much you exhale. Five seconds you inhale, three seconds you exhale – note it down.

Sometimes you feel very, very beautiful – note it down. What is the proportion of inhalation and exhalation, what is the length; is there any pause? Note it down. Feel your own breathing for seven days and make a note in your diary – how is it connected with your moods? Then you can sort it out. Whenever you want to drop a mood just use the opposite pattern, or if you want to bring on a mood then use the pattern.

Actors, knowingly, unknowingly, come to understand it – sometimes they have to be angry without being angry. So what do they do? – they have to create the breathing pattern. They may not be aware of it, but they start breathing as if they are angry, and soon the blood rushes in and poisons are released. Their eyes are red without being angry; they are in a subtle angry state without being angry. They have to make love without being in love; they have to show love without being in love. How do they do it? – they know a certain Yoga secret.

That's why I always say that a yogi can become the most perfect actor. He is! His stage is vast, that's all. He is acting – acting not on the stage, but on the stage of the world. He is an actor, he is not a doer. The difference is that he is taking part in a great drama, and he can remain a witness to it. He can remain aloof and detached.

When meditation produces extraordinary sense
perceptions,
the mind gains confidence and this helps
perseverance.

If you work out your breathing pattern, you will find the
secret keys of how to change the climate of the mind, how to
change the moods. If you work from both the poles, that will be
better. Try to be friendly toward the happy, indifferent toward
the evil, and also continue the change and transformation of
your breathing patterns. There will then be: ...*extraordinary
sense perceptions...*

If you have taken LSD, marijuana, hashish, you know that
...*extraordinary sense perceptions...* happen. You look at ordinary
things and they become extraordinary.

Aldous Huxley remembers that when he took LSD for the
first time he was sitting before an ordinary chair, and when he
went more and more deep with the drug, when he was "on," the
chair immediately started changing color. It became radiant; an
ordinary chair that he had never paid any attention to... It
became so beautiful, with many colors coming out of it, as if it
was made of diamonds. Such beautiful shapes and nuances that
he couldn't believe his eyes. What was happening? Later on he
remembered that this must have happened to Van Gogh because
he had painted a chair almost exactly the same.

A poet need not take LSD; he has an inbuilt system of
throwing LSD into the body. That is the difference between a
poet and an ordinary man. And that's why they say that a poet is
born, not made – he has an extraordinary body structure. The
chemicals in his body have a different quantity and quality to
them. That's why, where you don't see anything, he sees miracles. You see an ordinary tree, he sees something unbelievable.
You see ordinary clouds; a poet, if he is really a poet, never sees
anything ordinary – everything is extraordinarily beautiful.

The same happens to a yogi, because when you change your breathing and your attitudes, your body chemistry changes its pattern. You are going through a chemical transformation and your eyes become clear, a new perceptivity happens. The same old tree becomes absolutely new. You never knew its shade of green; it becomes radiant. All around you, the whole world takes a new shape. It is a paradise now, not the ordinary old rotten earth.

People around you are no longer the same. Your ordinary wife becomes the most beautiful woman. Everything changes with your clarity of perception. And when your eyes change, everything changes.

Patanjali says: *When meditation produces extraordinary sense perceptions, the mind gains confidence and this helps perseverance.* You become confident that you are on the right path. The world is becoming more and more beautiful, the ugliness is disappearing. The world is becoming more and more a harmony, the discord is disappearing. The world is becoming more and more "home," you are feeling more and more at ease in it. It is friendly – it is a love affair between you and the universe. You become more confident, and with your effort comes more perseverance.

Also, meditate on the inner light which is serene and beyond all sorrow.

This can be done only when you have attained a certain quality of perceptivity. You close your eyes, and find a flame – a beautiful flame near the heart, a blue light. But right now you cannot see it. It is there, it has been always there. When you die that blue light goes out of your body, but you cannot see it because when you were alive you couldn't see it.

Others will also not be able to see that something is going out, but Kirlian, a Russian has taken photographs with very sensitive films, and has found that when a person dies, something happens around the body. Some body energy, some light-like thing, leaves, goes and disappears into the cosmos. That light is always there. That is your center of being. It is near the heart with a blue flame.

When you have some perception, when your eyes are clear, you can see the beautiful world all around you. Close them and move nearer the heart; try to find what is there. First, you will feel darkness. It is just like when you come from the outside on a hot sunny day into a room and feel that everything is dark. But wait, let the eyes be attuned with the darkness, and soon you start seeing things in the house.

You have been outside for millions of lives. When you come in for the first time, nothing is there except darkness, emptiness. But wait. It will take a few days, even a few months, but just wait, close the eyes and look down into the heart. Suddenly, it happens one day; you see a light, a flame. Concentrate on that flame.

Nothing is more blissful than that. Nothing is more dancing, singing, musical, harmonious than that inner blue light within your heart. The more you concentrate, the more you become tranquil, silent, calm, collected. Then there is no darkness. When your heart is filled with light, the whole universe is filled with light. *Also, meditate on the inner light which is serene and beyond all sorrow.*

Also, meditate on one who has attained
desirelessness.

That too! Patanjali is giving you all the alternatives. A *vee-taraga*, one who has gone beyond all desires... Also meditate on him. Mahavira, Buddha, Patanjali – your own – Zarathustra, Mohammed, Christ or anybody you feel an affinity and love with. Meditate on one who has gone beyond desires. Meditate on your master, on your guru who has gone beyond desires. How will it help? – it helps because when you meditate on someone who has gone beyond desires, he becomes a magnetic force in you. You allow him to enter within you. He pulls you out of yourself. This becomes your availability to him.

If you meditate on someone who has gone beyond desires, sooner or later you will become like him because meditation makes you like the object of meditation itself. If you meditate on money, you will become just like money. Go and look at a miser; he no longer has a soul. He has only a bank balance, he has nothing inside. If you listen, you will just hear notes, dollars; you will not find any heart there.

Whatever you pay your attention to, you become like it. So be aware, and don't pay attention to something you would not like to become. Only pay attention to something you would like to become, because this is the beginning. The seed is sown with the attention, and soon it will become a tree.

You sow the seeds of hell, and when it becomes a tree you say, "Why am I so miserable?" You always pay attention to the wrong. You always look to that which is negative. You always pay attention to the fault, and you become faulty.

Don't pay attention to the fault. Pay attention to the beautiful. Why count the thorns? Why not see the flower? Why count the nights? Why not count the days? If you count the nights, there are two nights and only one day between the two. If you count the days, there are two days and only one night in between. It makes a lot of difference. Look at the light side if you want to become light. Look at the dark if you want to become dark.

Patanjali says: *Also, meditate on one who has attained desirelessness.* Seek a master, and surrender to him. Be attentive to him. Listen, watch, eat and drink him. Let him enter you, and allow your heart to be filled with him. Soon you will be on a journey because the object of attention ultimately becomes the goal of your life. And attention is a secret relationship. Through attention you become the object of your attention.

Krishnamurti goes on saying, "The observer becomes the observed." He is right; whatever you observe, you will become. So be alert! Beware! Don't observe something which you would not like to become because that is your goal; you are sowing the seeds.

Live near a *veetaraga*, a man who is beyond desires. Live near a man who has no more to fulfill here, who is fulfilled. His very fulfilledness will flood over you, and he will become a catalyst.

He will not do anything because a man who is beyond desires cannot do anything. Even he cannot help you because help is also a desire. Much help comes through him, but he doesn't help you. He becomes a catalyst without doing anything. If you allow him, he drops into your heart and his very presence crystallizes you.

Enough for today.

10

It's Difficult to Be Attracted to a Buddha

The first question:

Osho,
Do positive thoughts bring happenings too, like wishing
for enlightenment?

That is too much to ask from positive thoughts because enlightenment is beyond duality, it is neither negative nor positive. When both the polarities are dropped, it happens. With positive thoughts many things are possible – not enlightenment. You can be happy, but not blissful. Happiness comes and goes; the opposite always exists with it. When you are happy, just by the side, unhappiness is waiting for its own time. It is standing in the queue. When you are loving it is positive, but hate is waiting for its own time.

The positive cannot go beyond duality. It is good as far as it goes, but to ask enlightenment from it is too much. Never expect that. The negative has to be dropped to attain the positive. The positive has also to be dropped to attain the beyond. First drop the negative, then drop the positive. Nothing is left. That nothingness is enlightenment; there is no more mind.

The mind is either negative or positive; happy, unhappy;

loving, hateful; angry, compassionate. Day and night, birth and death – all belong to the mind. But *you* don't belong to mind. You are beyond it, encased in the mind but beyond it.

Enlightenment is not of the mind, it is of you. The realization that "I am not the mind" is enlightenment. If you remain negative, you remain in the valley part of the mind. If you are positive, you attain the peak part of the mind. But neither transcends the mental plane of your being. Drop both.

It is difficult to drop the positive; it is easy to drop the negative because it gives you misery. It is hell, you can drop it. But look at misfortune – you haven't even dropped that! You cling to the negative. You cling to misery as if it is a treasure. You cling to your unhappiness because it has become an old habit and you need something to cling to. Not finding anything, you cling to your hell. But remember, to drop the negative is easy however difficult it seems. Compared to the positive it is very easy because it is misery.

To drop the positive means to drop the happiness; to drop the positive means to drop all that looks like flowers, all that is beautiful. The negative is the ugly, the positive is the beautiful. The negative is death, the positive is life. But you can drop the negative, so take the first step. First feel the misery, how much it is given to you by the negative. Watch how the misery arises out of it, just watch and feel. The very feeling that the negative is creating the misery will become the dropping.

But the mind has a very deep trick. Whenever you are miserable it always says that someone else is responsible. Be alert, because if you are a victim of this trick, the negative can never be dropped. This is how the negative is hiding itself. You are angry; the mind says that someone has insulted you and that's why you are angry. That is not right. Someone may have insulted you, but that is just an excuse. You were already waiting to be angry. Anger was accumulating within you, otherwise someone would have insulted you and there would have been no anger.

The insult may become the visible cause of it, but it is not really the cause. You are boiling within. In fact, the person who insults you helps you. He helps you to bring your inner turmoil out and to be finished with it. You are in such bad shape that even an insult helps you. The enemy helps you because he helps to bring all the negativity out. At least you are unburdened for the time being.

The mind has this trick to always divert your consciousness toward the other. Immediately something goes wrong and you start looking for who has done this to you. In that looking you miss, and the real culprit is hiding behind.

Make it an absolute law that whenever something is wrong, immediately close your eyes and look for the real culprit. You will be able to see because it is a truth. It is a reality. It is true that you accumulate anger, that's why you become angry; it is true that you accumulate hate, that's why you feel hatred. The other is not a real cause. In Sanskrit they have two terms: one term is *karan*, the real cause, and the other term is *nimitta*, the unreal cause. The *nimitta*, the unreal cause which appears as the cause but is not, befools you. It has been befooling you for many, many lives.

Whenever you feel miserable, close your eyes immediately and go inside, because that is the right moment to catch the culprit red-handed; otherwise you will not be able to catch it. When the anger has disappeared, and you close your eyes, you will not find anything there. In a red-hot situation, don't miss the point. Make it a meditation.

You may start feeling that there is no method needed to drop the negative. The negative is so ugly, it is such a disease – how you carry it is amazing. Dropping is nothing; carrying is amazing. It has been a riddle for all the buddhas: how and why do you carry your diseases so lovingly? You are so careful with them that you are protecting all that is wrong. Protected, it gets deeper and deeper roots in you.

With the realization that it is your own negativity which

creates the problem, it falls by itself. When the negative mind falls by itself; there is a beauty. If you try to drop it, it will cling because the very effort to drop it shows that your understanding is not mature. All renunciation is immaturity; you are not ripe for it. That's why effort is needed to drop it. "I am carrying rubbish. Do I need any effort to drop it, except the understanding that this is rubbish? If I need any effort to drop it, that means I am supplementing my understanding with effort."

Understanding itself is not enough, that's why effort is needed. All those who have known, say effort is needed because your understanding is not there. It may be an intellectual thing, but you haven't really felt the situation, otherwise you simply drop it.

A snake crosses your path; you simply jump. There is no effort in the jump, you don't decide to jump. You don't make a logical syllogism within yourself that there is a snake, and wherever there is a snake there is danger; hence you must jump. You don't make a logical step-by-step syllogism. Even Aristotle will jump. Later on he can make the syllogism, but right now, the snake is there, and it doesn't bother about your logic – the whole situation is so dangerous. The very understanding that the situation is dangerous is enough.

For the negative to drop, no effort is needed, only understanding. Now the real problem arises: how to drop the positive? – because it is so beautiful. And for you who have not known the beyond, it is the ultimate in happiness – to be so happy. Look at a couple in love; look at their eyes, the way they walk hand in hand. They are happy. Tell them to drop this positive mind and they will think, "Are you crazy?" They have been waiting for this, and now it has happened. And here comes a buddha who says, "Drop it."

When somebody is succeeding, reaching higher and higher on the ladder, tell him to drop it. In his eyes, that is his very purpose. If he even thinks to drop it, he knows he will drop into misery because from the positive where will you move to?

You know only two possibilities: positive or negative. If you

drop the positive you move to the negative. That's why the negative has to be dropped first so that it is not possible to move to
the negative. Otherwise, if you drop the positive, the negative
enters immediately. If you are not happy, what will you be? –
unhappy! If you are not silent, what will you be? – a chatterbox!
Hence drop the negative first so one alternative is closed, and you
cannot move that way. Otherwise energy has a routine movement from positive to negative, from negative to positive. If the
negative exists, there is every possibility the moment you drop
the positive you will become the negative.

When you are not happy, you will be unhappy; you don't
know that there is a third possibility. The third possibility opens
only when the negative has been dropped and you drop the positive. For a moment there will be a pause. Energy cannot move
anywhere, not knowing where to move. The negative door is
closed, the positive has been closed. You will be for a moment...
And that moment will look like eternity. It will look very, very
long – never-ending.

For a moment you will be just in the middle, not knowing
what to do, or where to go. This moment will look like madness.
You are neither positive nor negative, then who are you? What
is your identity? Your identity, name and form drop with the
positive and negative. Suddenly you are nobody that you can recognize – just an energy phenomenon. And you cannot say how
you are feeling. There is no feeling. Bear this moment if you can
tolerate it; this is the greatest sacrifice, the greatest *tapascharya*,
and the whole of Yoga prepares you for this moment. Otherwise
the tendency will be to go somewhere, but not remain in this
vacuum; be positive, be negative, but don't remain in this vacuum.
You are nothing, as if you are disappearing. An abyss has opened,
and you are falling into it.

At this moment a master is needed who can say, "Wait! Don't
be afraid. I am here." This is just a lie, but you need it. Nobody
is there. Not even a master can be there because the master also

ends when your mind ends. Now you are absolutely alone, and to be alone is so fearsome, scary, deathlike, that somebody is needed to give you courage. It is only a one moment's question, and the lie helps.

I can tell you that because of their compassion toward you, all the buddhas have been liars. The master says, "Don't worry, I am here. Go ahead." You gain confidence, and take the jump. Just a moment's question, and everything hangs there. The whole of existence hangs there; the crossing point, the boiling point. If you take the step you are lost to the mind forever. There will be no positive, no negative ever again.

You can be scared. You can go back again and enter the negative or the positive which is cozy, comfortable, familiar. You were entering the unknown – this is the problem. First, the problem is how to drop the negative. A ripe understanding is needed. And that is the easiest thing, but you have not even done that.

The problem is then how to drop the positive, which is so beautiful and gives you such happiness. But if you drop the negative, if you become that ripe, you will have a second understanding, a second transformation, in which you will be able to see that if you don't drop the positive, the negative will come back. Then the positive loses all its positivity. It was positive only in comparison to the negative. Once the negative is thrown, even the positive becomes negative because now you can see all this happiness is momentary. When this moment is lost, where will you be? The negative will enter again.

Before the negative enters, drop it. Hell always comes through heaven. Heaven is just the gate; hell is the real place. Through heaven and the promise of heaven you enter hell. Hell is the real place; heaven is just the gate. How can you remain at the gate forever? Sooner or later you have to enter. Where will you go from the positive? Once the negative is dropped, you can see that the positive is just the other aspect of it – not really contrary, not opposite, but a conspiracy. They are both in conspiracy; they are together. When this understanding arises: that the positive has become the nega-tive, you can drop it.

In fact, to say that you can drop it is not good. It also drops. It has also become negative. You know that in this life there is nothing like happiness. Happiness is a trick for unhappiness to come in. It is just like the chicken and egg relationship. What is a chicken? – it is the way for the egg to come back. And what is an egg? – it is the way for the chicken to come back.

Positive and negative are not real opposites. They are like the chicken and egg, mother and child. They help each other and come from each other. But this understanding is possible only when the negative has been dropped. You can then drop the pos-itive. And you can stay in that transitory moment, which is the greatest moment in existence. You will never feel another moment so long – as if years are passing, because the vacuum… You lose all bearing; the whole of the past is lost, suddenly empty, not knowing where you are, who you are, what is happening.

This is the moment of madness. If you try to return from this moment you will always remain mad. Many people go mad through meditation. From this moment they fall back, and now there is nothing to fall back to because the positive-negative has been dropped. They no longer exist; the house is no longer there. Once you leave the house it disappears. It depended on you; it is not a separate entity.

The mind is not a separate entity; it depends on you. Once you leave it, it is no longer there. You cannot come back, you cannot fall back to it. That is the state of madness. You have not attained transcendence, and you come back and look for the mind – it is no longer there. The house has disappeared. To be in this state is very, very painful. For the first time there is real anguish. Hence the master, the need for the master, who will not allow you to come back, who will force you to go ahead because once you turn back it will take so much effort to bring you to that point again. For many lives you may miss it because now there is no mind to even understand.

In Sufism, this state is called the state of a *mast* – the state of a madman. This state is really difficult to understand because the man is and is not – both. He laughs and weeps together. He has lost all orientation, he doesn't know what weeping is or what laughing is. Is there any contradiction? He beats himself and enjoys himself, and celebrates beating himself. He doesn't know what he is doing, whether it is harmful or not. He becomes completely dependent. He becomes like a small child; he has to be taken care of.

If someone goes into meditation without a master, this can be the outcome. With a master, the master will be the barrier. He will be just standing behind you and will not allow you to go back. He will become a rock. And, finding no way to go back, you will have to take the jump. Nobody can take it for you, nobody can be with you at that moment. Once you take this jump you have transcended all dualities. Negative, positive, both gone – this is enlightenment.

I talk about the positive so that you can drop the negative. Once you drop the negative you are trapped. Then the positive has to be dropped. Each step leads to another in such a way that if you take the first step the second is bound to come. It is a chain. In fact, only the first has to be taken, all else follows. If you understand – the first is the last. The beginning is the end: the alpha is the omega.

The second question:

Osho,
Please describe the developmental gap between the man of spiritual experience who has already attained a certain degree of higher awareness – even certain psychic skills and capacities – and the fully enlightened being, the living buddha.

This is the difference: a man who has become absolutely positive is the man of spiritual attainment. The person who has become absolutely negative... When I say absolutely negative, I mean ninety-nine percent negative because absolute negativity is not possible. Neither is absolute positivity possible; the other is needed. The quantity can change, the degrees differ.

The man who is ninety-nine percent negative and one percent positive is the most fallen of men, what Christians call the sinner – one percent positive. That too is needed only to help his ninety-nine percent negativity. He is negative in everything. Whatever you say, no is the only response; whatever existence asks, no is the only response. The atheist is one who cannot say yes to anything; who has become incapable of saying yes, and cannot trust. This man suffers hell. And because he says no to everything, he becomes a no, a yawning no; anger, violence, suppression, sadness, all together – he becomes hell personified.

It is difficult to find such a man because it is difficult to be such a man. It is very difficult to live ninety-nine percent in hell. But just to explain it to you, I am saying: "This is the mathematical possibility that one can become if one tries. You will not find such a man anywhere. Even a Hitler is not that destructive." The whole energy becomes destructive, not only of others, but of oneself also. The whole attitude is suicidal. When a person commits suicide, what is he saying? – he is saying no to life through his death. He is saying no to God; he is saying: "You cannot create me. I will destroy myself."

Sartre, one of the great thinkers of this age, says that suicide is the only freedom – freedom from God. Why freedom from God? – because there is no freedom. You don't have any freedom to create yourself. Whenever you are, you find yourself already created. Birth you cannot take, that is not your freedom. But Sartre says, "You can commit death. That is your freedom." At least you can say one definite thing to God: "I am free." This man who always lives near the abyss of suicide is the last, the greatest sinner.

In existentialism, which Sartre preaches, these words have become very meaningful: anguish, boredom, sadness. They have to become meaningful because this man will live in anguish, boredom. One percent positivity is needed. He will say yes to boredom, suicide, anguish. For this much he has a need to say yes. This is the modern man, who is coming nearer and nearer to this lost soul. This is the sinner, the fallen.

The spiritual man exists on the other peak, ninety-nine percent positive, one percent negative. He says yes to everything. He has only one no, and that no is against no, that's all. Otherwise he is yes. But because a total yes cannot exist, he has a need to say no.

This man attains many things because the positive mind can give you millions of things. This man will be happy, serene, collected, calm and quiet; this mind will flower and give all its positive qualities to him. He will have certain powers; he can read your thoughts, he can heal you. His blessing will become a force. Just by being near him, you will be benefited. In subtle ways he is a blessing.

All the *siddhis* – all the powers that Yoga talks about and Patanjali talks about later on – will be easy to him. He will be a man of miracles, his touch will be magical. Anything is possible because he has a ninety-nine percent positive mind. Positivity is a force, a power. He will be very powerful, but still he is not enlightened. It will be easier for you to think of this man as enlightened than to think of an enlightened man as enlightened, because the enlightened man simply goes beyond you. You cannot understand him, he becomes incomprehensible.

In fact, an enlightened man has no power because he has no mind. He is not miraculous. He has no mind, he cannot do anything. He is the ultimate in non-doing. Miracles can happen around him, but they happen because of your mind, not because of him; that is the difference. A spiritual man can do miracles, not an enlightened man. Miracles are possible, but they will happen because of you, not because of him. Your trust, your faith will do the miracle because you become the positive mind in that moment.

Like Jesus says…

A woman touched his gown; he was moving in a crowd, and the woman was so poor and so old she never believed that Jesus would bless her, so she thought it would be good to be in the crowd and when Jesus passes, just to touch his gown. "It is *his* gown, and the very touch is enough. I am so poor and so old, who will care, who will bother about me? There will be many people, and Jesus will be interested in them." So she simply touched his gown.

Jesus looked back, and the woman said, "I am healed!"

Jesus said, "It is because of your faith. I haven't done anything, you have done it to yourself."

Many miracles happen, but the man who is enlightened cannot do anything. The mind is the doer, the doer of all. When the mind is no longer there, there are happenings, but no more doings. In fact, an enlightened man, is no more. He exists as a non-entity, as an emptiness. He is a shrine – empty. You can enter him, but you will not meet him. He has gone beyond the polarities. He is a great beyond. You will be lost in him, but you cannot find him.

A man of spiritual powers is still in the world. He is your polar opposite. You feel helpless, he feels powerful. You feel unhealthy, he can heal you. It's bound to be so. You are ninety-nine percent negative and he is ninety-nine percent positive. The very meeting is between impotence and power. Positivity is power; negativity is impotence. You will be very impressed by such a man, and that becomes the danger for him; the more you are impressed by him, the more his ego strengthens. With a negative man, the ego can't be very strong because the ego needs positive power.

That's why you can find very, very humble people in sinners, but never in saints. Saints are always egotistic. They are somebody – powerful, chosen, elite, messengers of God, prophets. They are somebody. A sinner is humble – afraid of himself, he moves carefully; he knows who he is. Many times it has happened that a sinner has taken a direct jump and become enlightened, but it has never been so easy for a man of spiritual power because the very power becomes the hindrance.

Patanjali talks much about it. He has a complete section of sutras devoted to *vibhuti pada*, to this dimension of power. And he has written the whole part just to make you aware not to become a victim of it because the ego is very subtle. It is such a subtle phenomenon and such a deceptive force that wherever there is power, it sucks on it. This ego is a sucking phenomenon. So in the world the ego finds politics, prestige, power, wealth. Then it feels like somebody. You are a president of a country or a prime minister – you are somebody. Or you have millions of dollars – you are somebody. The ego is strengthened.

The game remains the same because the positive is not out of the world. The positive is within the world – better than the negative, but there is more danger. A man who feels he's great because he is a prime minister, a president, a very rich man, also knows that he cannot carry these riches beyond death. But a man who feels powerful because of psychic forces such as ESP, thought reading, clairvoyance, clairaudience, astral traveling, healing, feels more egotistic. He knows he can carry these powers beyond death. And yes, they can be carried, because it is the mind that is reborn, and these forces belong to the mind.

Wealth belongs to the body, not to the mind; you cannot carry it. A political power belongs to the body. When you are dead you are nobody. But these forces, these spiritual powers belong to the mind, and the mind moves from one body to another. It is carried. From the very beginning you will be born in the next life as a charismatic child, you will have a magnetic force in you. Hence, more attraction; hence, more danger.

Remember, don't try to become spiritual. The spiritual is against the material, just as the negative is against the positive. In fact, they are not opposites. The quality of both is the same. One is superior and subtle; the other is gross and inferior, but both are the same. Don't be deceived by spiritual powers. Whenever spiritual powers start arising in you, you have to be more alert than ever – they *will* arise. As you meditate more, the mind will become refined. When the mind is refined, the seeds which you have been carrying will always start sprouting. Now the soil is ready, the season has come and those flowers are beautiful.

When you can touch somebody and they are healed immediately, it is difficult to resist the temptation. When you can be of so much benefit to people, when you can become a great servant, it is very difficult to resist the temptation. Temptations arise immediately and you rationalize them because you are doing it in the service of the people. But look within; through serving people the ego arises, and then the greatest barrier is there.

Materialism is not such a great barrier. Just like the negative mind it is not a great barrier to drop. It is suffering. The positive is difficult to drop, spirituality is difficult to drop. You can drop the body easily; the real problem is to drop the mind. But unless you drop both the material and the spiritual – neither this nor that – unless you go beyond both, you are not enlightened.

In fact, an enlightened man is simply very, very ordinary. He has nothing special, and that is the specialty. He is so ordinary that you can pass him by on the street. You cannot pass by a spiritual man. He will bring a wave all around him; he will be energy. If he passes you on the street you will be simply bathed by him – attracted like a magnet.

But you can pass a buddha – if you don't know that he is a buddha, you will not know – but you cannot pass a Rasputin. A Rasputin is not a bad man; a Rasputin is a spiritual man. You cannot pass by a Rasputin. The moment you see him you are magnetized. You will follow him for the whole of your life. This happened to the czar. Once he saw this man he became his slave. He had tremendous power. He would come like a strong wind; it was difficult not to be attracted by him.

It is difficult to be attracted to a buddha. Many times you can pass him by. He is so simple and ordinary, and that is the extra-ordinariness because now the negative and the positive are both lost; he is no longer under the electric realm – he exists. He exists like a rock, like a tree; he exists like a sky. If you allow him he can enter you; he will not even knock at your door. No, he will not even be that aggressive. He is a very, very silent phenomenon. He is a nothingness.

But this is the greatest thing to achieve because only he knows what existence is, only he knows what being is. With the negative and the positive you know the mind; the negative is impotent, the positive is powerful.

Never try to be spiritual. It will happen automatically, you need not try it. And when it happens, remain detached.

In the past there were many, many stories…

Buddha had a cousin-brother, his name was Devadatta. He had taken initiation from Buddha. He was a cousin-brother and, of course, deep down jealous – a very powerful man, like Rasputin. Soon he started gathering his own following, and started saying to people, "I can do many things and this Buddha cannot do anything."

Again and again followers came to Buddha and said, "Devadatta is trying to create a separate sect, and he says that he is more pow-erful." He was right, but his power belonged to the positive mind. He made many efforts to kill Buddha. On one occasion he made an elephant mad. When I say that he made an elephant mad, I mean that he used his positive power and it was such a strong phenomenon that the elephant became intoxicated, he rushed about madly, and tore down many trees. Devadatta was very happy because Buddha was sitting just behind the trees, and the elephant was going mad – just a mad energy. But when the elephant came near Buddha, he looked at him sitting silently in deep meditation... Devadatta was puzzled.

What happened? – when there is emptiness, everything is absorbed. Emptiness has no limits; the madness was absorbed. Not that Buddha had done anything – he is just a vacuum. The elephant came rushing toward him, lost his energy and became silent. He became so silent that it is said that Devadatta tried many times, but he could not make that elephant mad again.

The enlightened man is not a man at all, that is one thing; he is not at all, that is another thing. He appears to be there, but he is not. You see his body, but not him. The more you search for him, the possibility of finding him is less. In the very search you will be lost. He has become the universal. The spiritual man is still an individual.

So remember, your mind will try to become spiritual. Your mind has a hankering to be more powerful, to be somebody in this world of nobodies. Be alert to it. Even if much benefit can be carried out through it, it is dangerous. The benefit is only on the surface. Deep down you are killing yourself, and soon it will be lost and you will fall into the negative again. It is a certain energy; you can lose it. You can make use of it, then it is gone.

Hindus have a very scientific category; that categorization exists nowhere else. In the West they think in terms of hell and heaven – just two things. Hindus think in three categories: hell, heaven and *moksha*. It is difficult to translate the third into Western languages because no category exists. We call it liberation, but it is not. It gives the feeling, just the fragrance of it, but it is not exactly the same.

Heaven and hell are there; the third is not there. Hell is the negative mind in its perfection; heaven is the positive mind in its perfection. But where is the beyond? In India they say that if you are a spiritualist, when you die you will be born in a heaven. You will live there for millions of years, happy, absolutely enjoying everything, but you will have to fall back to the earth again. With your energy lost, you will have to come back. You earned a particular energy, then you used it. You will fall back again to the same situation.

So in India they say, "Don't seek heaven." Even if you will be happy for millions of years, that happiness is not going to be forever. You will lose it, you will fall back. It is not worth the effort. Hindus call them *devatas*, those who live in heaven – the people who reside in heaven.

They are not *muktas*, they are not enlightened, but they are positive; they have reached the peak of their positive energy, the mind energy. They can fly in the sky; they can move from one point of space to another immediately with no time gap. The moment they desire something, it is fulfilled immediately with no time gap. Here you desire, there it is fulfilled. They have beautiful bodies, forever young, that never become old. Their bodies are golden; they live in golden cities with young women, and they are continuously happy – with wine, women and dancing. In fact, only one problem exists there – that is boredom. They get bored. That is the only negative – one percent negative, and ninety-nine percent happy. They simply get bored, and sometimes even try to come onto earth. They can come; they can come and try to mingle with human beings just to break the boredom.

But finally they fall back, as if finally coming out of a dream, a beautiful dream, that's all. According to Hindus, heaven is a dream, a beautiful dream. Hell is also a dream, a nightmare. Both are dreams because both belong to the mind. Remember this definition: all that belongs to the mind is a dream. Positive, negative, whatever – the mind is a dream. To go beyond the dream, to awake, is to become enlightened.

It is difficult to say anything about the enlightened man because he cannot be defined. A definition is possible if there is some limitation. He is as vast as a sky; a definition is not possible. The only way to know an enlightened man is to become enlightened. The spiritual man can be defined, he has his limitations; there is no difficulty in defining him within the mind.

When we come to *vibhuti pada*, to Patanjali's sutras about *siddhis*, powers, we will see that he can be defined completely. In the West scientific research is going on, which they call "psychic" research. Psychic societies exist all over the world. Many universities now have labs for psychic research. Sooner or later what Patanjali says will be scientifically categorized and proved. In a way it is good; it is good because you will then be able to know that this is something of the mind which can even be examined by mechanical devices, categorized and finished. You cannot have any glimpse of enlightenment through any mechanical device. It is not a phenomenon of the body or of the mind. It is very elusive, mysterious.

Remember one thing: never try to gain any spiritual powers. Even if they come by themselves on your path, drop them immediately. Don't move in their company and don't listen to their tricks. They will say, "What is wrong in it? You can help others. You can become a great benefactor." But don't become that. Simply say, "I am not in search of power and nobody can help anybody." You can become an entertainment, but you cannot help anybody.

How can you help anybody? Everybody moves according to his own karmas. In fact, if a man of spiritual power touches you and your disease disappears, what is happening? – deep down your disease was going to disappear; your karmas were fulfilled. It is just an excuse that it disappeared by the touch of a spiritual man. It was going to disappear – because you did something, that's why it was there. And now the time has come… You cannot help anybody in any way. There is only one help – that you become that which you would like everybody to become. You simply become that. Your very presence, not your doing, will be helpful.

What does Buddha do? – he is simply there, available, like a river. Those who are thirsty will come. Even if a river tries to satisfy your thirst, if you are not ready, it is impossible. Even with a river that is flowing, if you don't open your mouth, and bow down to receive the water, you will remain thirsty. This is what is happening; the river is flowing and you are sitting on the bank thirsty. The ego will always remain thirsty, whatever it attains. Ego is thirst. Satiety is of the soul, not of the ego.

The third question:

Osho,
What is the secret to how you can work on so many of us at the same time?

I don't work at all! I am simply here. It doesn't make any difference how many of you are around me. If I work, then, of course, how can I work on so many at the same time? My work is of a different quality; in fact, it is not work. I have to use these words because of you. I am simply here. Things will happen if you are also here. I am available. If you are also available, things will happen by themselves; nothing needs to be done.

A meeting is needed of two availabilities, of two presences; then things happen by themselves. What do you do when you plant a seed in the earth? What do you do? – there is just the meeting of the seed and the earth and things happen by themselves, just like that.

I am here. If you are also here... And that is the problem; you may seem to be here and you may not be here – then nothing happens. I am here. If you are also here, things happen by themselves – just like that. I am not doing anything, otherwise I will get tired of you. I am never tired because I am not doing anything. You cannot tire me, I am not bored – otherwise, I will be bored. So many of you are even bored with yourselves.

It happened in a Jewish community…

A rabbi threatened to leave; the holy days were nearing and the trustees were worried what to do. It would be difficult at that moment to find a new rabbi, and the old one was adamant. So they tried to persuade him to stay. They sent a delegation of three trustees, and told them to persuade him to stay in any way they could. If he wants more salary, "Say okay," or tell him, "Just stay here at least a few more weeks and then you can leave. We will be able to find…" So they went, and tried in every way to persuade him to stay. They said to him, "We love and respect you. Why are you leaving?"

The rabbi replied, "If only five people like you were here, I would have remained!"

They felt flattered because he had said, "If only five people like you were here, I would have remained." They felt very good and said, "But it will not be very difficult; we are three, two more can be found."

The rabbi said, "It is not difficult; that is the problem. There are two hundred people like you here, and it is too much!"

You are bored with yourself. Look in the mirror – you are bored with your own face. And so many of you are here, I must be bored to death! You go on bringing the same problems to me every day, but I am never bored because I am not working. This is not work at all. You may call it love, but not work – and love is never bored. You can bring the same problems to me a thousand times – again and again – and there are not many problems. I have been watching thousands of people. The same problems repeat themselves again and again. Your problems are just like seven days of the week, not more than that. Monday comes again, Tuesday comes again… It goes on and on. But I am not even a little bit bored because I am not working. If you are working, then of course it is very, very difficult. That's why I can work – because I am not working.

There are many of you, and the only thing required is from you, not from me. You may be tired of me someday, that's possible. You may try to escape from me, that's possible. Only one thing is required of you; if you can do that, there is no need to do anything either on my part or on your part. That thing is your availability; be here and now, and it makes no difference whether you are here in this city, in this ashram, or on the other side of the world.

The seeds will sprout if you are available. I am available everywhere; that is not the point. Even when I am not in this body I will be available. But it will be more and more difficult for you because you are not available even when I am in this body, here and now just talking to you. You are not listening! You are hearing of course, but not listening. You are looking at me, but not at me. Look at me! It is not work. It is just a love that is available, and through love everything is possible – every transformation.

The fourth question:

Osho,
You mentioned that love is a need. Why is this essential
need always so hard to fulfill for most people?

Many things are involved. One thing being that society is against love because love is the greatest bond, and love separates you from society. Two lovers become a world in themselves; they don't bother about anybody. Hence, society is against, and doesn't want you to love. Marriage – granted, but not love because once you love a person you become a separate world in yourself. You don't bother about what is happening to others in the world. You simply forget them. You create a private world of your own.

Love is such a creative force it becomes a universe. You start moving around your own center, and society cannot tolerate this. Your parents cannot tolerate your love because if you are in love you forget them completely, as if they never existed. They exist on the margin, somewhere very distant. How can they allow you to love? They will make arrangements for your marriage, and that will be their arrangement. You will exist as part of the family.

Mulla Nasruddin fell in love with a woman. He came home very happy and when the family were eating their supper together he said, "I have decided who to marry."

The father said immediately, "This is not possible. Impossible! I cannot allow it because the girl's family have not left her a single paisa. She is bankrupt. Better girls are available with better dowries. Don't be foolish."

The mother said, "That girl? We could never have imagined that you could be so stupid – because she never does anything except read silly novels. She is of no use; she cannot cook, she cannot clean the house. Look at the dirty house she lives in!"

And so on, and so forth. Every member of the family rejected the girl according to his own judgments. The younger brother said, "I won't agree because of her nose – the nose is so ugly." And everybody had his or her opinion.

Then Nasruddin said, "But there is one thing that the girl has which we don't have."

They all asked in chorus, "What is that?"

He replied, "The family; she doesn't have a family. That is one beautiful thing about her."

Parents are against love. From the very beginning, they train you in such a way that you don't fall in love because love will go against the family, and the society is nothing but a greater family. Love goes against society, civilization, religion, priests. Love is such an involvement, such a total commitment, it goes against everybody. And everybody has an investment in you.

No, it cannot be allowed. You have been trained not to love – that's the difficulty. This difficulty comes from the society, culture, civilization, that is all around you. But this is not the greatest difficulty. There is still one that comes from you and which is even greater, and that is: love needs a surrender. Love needs you to drop the ego.

You are also against love. You would like love to become a celebration of your ego; you would like love to become an ornament for your ego. You would like love to follow you like a dog, but love never follows anybody like a dog. Love needs you in a total surrender. It is not that the woman surrenders to the man or that the man surrenders to the woman, no; both surrender to love. Love is a god. Love is really the only god, and it requires you – both the lovers – to be completely surrendered to it.

Lovers, what are they doing? The husband tries to get the wife to surrender to him and the wife tries to get the husband to surrender to her. How can love be possible? Love is something else – both should surrender to it, and both should disappear into it. This becomes the greatest barrier; you cannot love because of "you." These two things together, and love becomes impossible. If love becomes impossible, life becomes impossible. If love becomes impossible, prayer becomes impossible. If love becomes impossible, God becomes impossible. All that is beautiful grows out of love. The soil of love is a must, otherwise you will remain crippled. You try to complement and supplement it in other ways, but nothing can supplement it, no substitute exists.

You can go on praying, but your prayer will lack the grace that comes when one has loved. How can you "do" prayer? Your prayer will be just rubbish, a verbal phenomenon. You will say something to God, talk to him and go to sleep, but it will lack the essential quality. How can you pray when you have not loved? Prayer comes through the heart, and your heart has remained closed so the prayer comes from the head, and the head cannot become the heart.

So all over the world people go on praying. They are just gestures; the essential is not there. The prayer is without roots. Love

THE HEART OF YOGA

prepares the soil. It prepares the ground for the prayer to come. Prayer is nothing but a higher love, a love which transcends individuals, a love which goes to the whole, not to the part. But you need to learn with the part.

You cannot just jump into the ocean. You need to learn to swim in a swimming pool. Love is a swimming pool where you are protected and can learn. Then you can go to the seas, to the wild seas. You cannot jump directly into the wild seas. If you take the jump you will be in danger – that's not possible. Love is a small swimming pool, there are only two people. The whole world is very small... It is possible to enter each other. But even there you are afraid. In a swimming pool you are afraid: "I may go, I may be drowned." What to say about the ocean? Love is the first grounding, the first readiness to take a greater jump. I teach you love and I tell you that whatever is at stake, don't bother; sacrifice it – prestige, wealth, family, society, culture. Whatever is at stake, don't bother. Be a gambler because there is nothing like love. If you lose everything, you lose nothing if you gain love. If you lose love, whatever you gain you gain nothing. Be aware of these two things.

Society will not help you; it is against love. Love is an antisocial force, and society tries to suppress it. Then you can be used in many ways. For example, if you are really in love you cannot be made into a soldier, you cannot be sent to war. That's impossible because you don't bother about it; you say, "What's a country? What is this patriotism? Nonsense!" Love is such a beautiful flower; patriotism, nationalism, country, the flag, all look like nonsense to one who has known. You have tasted the real thing.

Society tries to divert you. The real thing should not be tasted. You are hankering for love, and your love can be diverted in any direction. It can become patriotism, you go and become a martyr. You are a fool because you are wasting yourself! You can go and die, your love has been diverted. If you don't love, your love can become a love of money. You become an accumulator, a hoarder. Your family will be happy, you are doing beautifully.

You are simply committing suicide. The family is happy because you are accumulating so much wealth. They missed their life; now they are forcing you to miss yours. They do it in such a loving way that you also cannot say no. They make you feel guilty. If you hoard money they are happy. But how can a man who loves hoard? It is difficult. A lover is never a hoarder. A lover shares, distributes, goes on giving. A lover cannot hoard.

When love is not there you become miserly because you are afraid. You don't have the shelter of love, so you need some shelter. Wealth becomes the substitute. Society also wants you to hoard because how is wealth to be created if everyone becomes a lover? Society will be very, very rich, but rich in a totally different way. It may be poor materially, but it will be rich spiritually.

But that richness is not visible. Society needs visible wealth; the whole world of religion, society, culture is in a conspiracy because you have only one energy – that is love energy. If it moves rightly into love, it cannot be forced to move anywhere else. If you don't love, your very missing of it may become a research into science.

Freud had many glimpses of truth; he was really a rare man, and had many insights. He said that whenever you penetrate anything, it is penetrating the woman. If you are not allowed to have a woman, you will try to penetrate something else. You may penetrate toward being a prime minister of a country.

You will never find lovers within politicians; they will always sacrifice love for their power. Scientists will never be lovers because if they become lovers they relax. They need a tension, a constant obsession. Love relaxes; a constant obsession is not possible. They go madly to their laboratories. They are obsessed, possessed; they work night and day.

History knows that whenever a country's love-need is fulfilled, the country becomes weak. It can be defeated. So the love-need should not be fulfilled; then the country is dangerous because everybody is a maniac and ready to fight. With the slightest provocation, everybody is ready to fight. If the love-need is fulfilled, who bothers? Just think, if the whole country has been in love and somebody attacks, we will say to them: "Okay, you can also come and be here. Why bother? We are so happy, you can come as well. The country is vast; you can be here and be happy. And if you want to be the rulers, be the rulers. Nothing is wrong; so far so good. You take the responsibility. It's good!"

But when the love-need is not fulfilled, you are always ready to fight. Just remember, just try to watch your own mind. If you have not loved your woman for a few days, you are constantly feeling irritated. You love and relax. The irritation goes, and you feel so good that you can forgive. A lover can forgive everything. Love has been such a blessing, he can forgive all that is wrong.

No, leaders won't allow you to love because soldiers cannot be created. Where will you find warmongers, maniacs, mad people who would like to destroy? Love is creativity. If the love-need is fulfilled you would like to create, not to destroy. The whole political structure will fall down. If you love, the whole family structure will be totally different. If you love, the economy and the economics will be different. In fact, if love is allowed, the whole world will take a totally different shape. It cannot be allowed because this structure has its investments. Every structure pushes itself onward, and if you are crushed it doesn't bother.

The whole of humanity is crushed, and the chariot of civilization goes on and on. Realize this, watch this, be aware of this. Love is so simple, nothing is more simple than that. Drop all that society needs; remember your inner needs. That is not going against society. You are simply trying to enrich your own life. You are not here to fulfill anybody else's expectations; you are here for your own thing, for your own fulfillment.

Make that the primary, the base, and don't bother about other things. There are mad people all around you, and they will push you toward madness. No need to go against society; just drop out of its investments, that's all.

You need not become rebellious, a revolutionary, because that too is coming to the same thing again. If your love is not fulfilled you will become a revolutionary because that too is a destruction in disguise. And then comes the real problem: dropping your own ego. Love needs total surrender.

Allow this to happen, because there is nothing else which can happen to you. You will be wasted if you don't allow it to happen. If you allow it to happen, many more things become possible. One thing leads to another. Love always leads to prayer, that's why Jesus insists that God is love.

Enough for today.

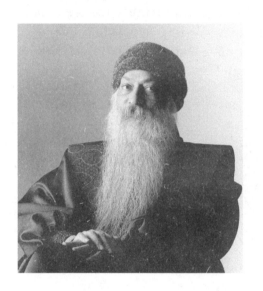

About Osho

Osho's unique contribution to the understanding of who we are defies categorization. Mystic and scientist, a rebellious spirit whose sole interest is to alert humanity to the urgent need to discover a new way of living. To continue as before is to invite threats to our very survival on this unique and beautiful planet.

His essential point is that only by changing ourselves, one individual at a time, can the outcome of all our "selves" – our societies, our cultures, our beliefs, our world – also change. The doorway to that change is meditation.

Osho the scientist has experimented and scrutinized all the approaches of the past and examined their effects on the modern human being and responded to their shortcomings by creating a new starting point for the hyperactive 21ˢᵗ Century mind: OSHO Active Meditations.

Once the agitation of a modern lifetime has started to settle, "activity" can melt into "passivity," a key starting point of real meditation. To support this next step, Osho has transformed the ancient "art of listening" into a subtle contemporary methodology: the OSHO Talks. Here words become music, the listener discovers who is listening, and the awareness moves from what is being heard to the individual doing the listening. Magically, as silence arises, what needs to be heard is understood directly, free from the distraction of a mind that can only interrupt and interfere with this delicate process.

These thousands of talks cover everything from the individual quest for meaning to the most urgent social and political issues facing society today. Osho's books are not written but are transcribed from audio and video recordings of these extem-poraneous talks to international audiences. As he puts it, "So remember: whatever I am saying is not just for you...I am talking also for the future generations."

Osho has been described by *The Sunday Times* in London as one of the "1000 Makers of the 20th Century" and by American author Tom Robbins as "the most dangerous man since Jesus Christ." *Sunday Mid-Day* (India) has selected Osho as one of ten people – along with Gandhi, Nehru and Buddha – who have changed the destiny of India.

About his own work Osho has said that he is helping to create the conditions for the birth of a new kind of human being. He often characterizes this new human being as "Zorba the Buddha" – capable both of enjoying the earthy pleasures of a Zorba the Greek and the silent serenity of a Gautama the Buddha.

Running like a thread through all aspects of Osho's talks and meditations is a vision that encompasses both the timeless wisdom of all ages past and the highest potential of today's (and tomorrow's) science and technology.

Osho is known for his revolutionary contribution to the science of inner transformation, with an approach to meditation that acknowledges the accelerated pace of contemporary life. His unique OSHO Active Meditations™ are designed to first release the accumulated stresses of body and mind, so that it is then easier to take an experience of stillness and thought-free relaxation into daily life.

Two autobiographical works by the author are available:
Autobiography of a Spiritually Incorrect Mystic,
St Martins Press, New York (book and eBook)
Glimpses of a Golden Childhood,
OSHO Media International, Pune, India (book and eBook)

OSHO International Meditation Resort

Each year the Meditation Resort welcomes thousands of people from more than 100 countries. The unique campus provides an opportunity for a direct personal experience of a new way of living – with more awareness, relaxation, celebration and creativity. A great variety of around-the-clock and around-the-year program options are available. Doing nothing and just relaxing is one of them!

All of the programs are based on Osho's vision of "Zorba the Buddha" – a qualitatively new kind of human being who is able *both* to participate creatively in everyday life *and* to relax into silence and meditation.

Location
Located 100 miles southeast of Mumbai in the thriving modern city of Pune, India, the OSHO International Meditation Resort is a holiday destination with a difference. The Meditation Resort is spread over 28 acres of spectacular gardens in a beautiful tree-lined residential area.

OSHO Meditations
A full daily schedule of meditations for every type of person includes both traditional and revolutionary methods, and particularly the OSHO Active Meditations™. The daily meditation program takes place in what must be the world's largest meditation hall, the OSHO Auditorium.

OSHO Multiversity
Individual sessions, courses and workshops cover everything from creative arts to holistic health, personal transformation, relationship and life transition, transforming meditation into a

lifestyle for life and work, esoteric sciences, and the "Zen" approach to sports and recreation. The secret of the OSHO Multiversity's success lies in the fact that all its programs are combined with meditation, supporting the understanding that as human beings we are far more than the sum of our parts.

OSHO Basho Spa
The luxurious Basho Spa provides for leisurely open-air swimming surrounded by trees and tropical green. The uniquely styled, spacious Jacuzzi, the saunas, gym, tennis courts…all these are enhanced by their stunningly beautiful setting.

Cuisine
A variety of different eating areas serve delicious Western, Asian and Indian vegetarian food – most of it organically grown especially for the Meditation Resort. Breads and cakes are baked in the resort's own bakery.

Night life
There are many evening events to choose from – dancing being at the top of the list! Other activities include full-moon meditations beneath the stars, variety shows, music performances and meditations for daily life.

Facilities
You can buy all of your basic necessities and toiletries in the Galleria. The Multimedia Gallery sells a large range of OSHO media products. There is also a bank, a travel agency and a Cyber Café on-campus. For those who enjoy shopping, Pune provides all the options, ranging from traditional and ethnic Indian products to all of the global brand-name stores.

Accommodation
You can choose to stay in the elegant rooms of the OSHO

Guesthouse, or for longer stays on campus you can select one of the OSHO Living-In programs. Additionally there is a plentiful variety of nearby hotels and serviced apartments.

www.osho.com/meditationresort
www.osho.com/guesthouse
www.osho.com/livingin

For More Information

www.**OSHO**.com

a comprehensive multi-language website including a magazine, OSHO Books, OSHO Talks in audio and video formats, the OSHO Library text archive in English and Hindi and extensive information about OSHO Meditations. You will also find the program schedule of the OSHO Multiversity and information about the OSHO International Meditation Resort.

http://OSHO.com/AllAboutOSHO
http://OSHO.com/Resort
http://OSHO.com/Shop
http://www.youtube.com/OSHO
http://www.Twitter.com/OSHO
http://www.facebook.com/pages/OSHO.International

To contact OSHO International Foundation:
www.osho.com/oshointernational,
oshointernational@oshointernational.com